HELPING OTHERS IN
•CRISIS•

FAMILIES OF HANDICAPPED CHILDREN

MARION DUCKWORTH

David C. Cook Publishing Co.
Elgin, Illinois—Weston, Ontario

David C. Cook Publishing Co.
Elgin, Illinois—Weston, Ontario
Families of Handicapped Children
© 1988 David C. Cook Publishing Co.

Scripture quotations, unless otherwise noted, are from the *Holy Bible: New International Version.* © 1978 by the New York International Bible Society. Used by permission of Zondervan Bible Publishers.

Published by David C. Cook Publishing Co.
850 N. Grove Ave., Elgin, IL 60120
Cable address: DCCOOK
Designed by Christopher Patchel and Michael Letwenko
Illustrated by Michael Letwenko
Printed in the United States of America
Library of Congress Catalog Card Number 88-70184

ISBN: 1-55513-084-4

Thanks to Ruth McEwen, who made herself available to me, and whose expertise and insights have been extremely valuable. Credit goes also to the National Information Center for Handicapped Children and Youth, as well as to parents, organizations and associations for handicapped people, and to Charlotte Thompson, M.D., for her book, *Raising a Handicapped Child* (Morrow, 1986). Thanks also to the many others who have worked hard to make information about handicapped persons available. I have tried to give credit where I can, but there are so many that it is impossible to mention everyone. Please know that I am grateful to you all.

—To Ruth McEwen

CONTENTS

I MET DORIS ON A SUMMER AFTERNOON. WE WERE DOING WHAT most good New York City apartment-dwelling mothers did then—supervising our children while they got fresh air and exercise outdoors in the neighborhood.

I had two sons; Doris had one. My three-year-old was riding his tricycle up and down the sidewalk while his baby brother slept in his carriage. Doris's nine-year-old kept riding his over-sized trike while we talked. Unspoken in the back of my mind while we made conversation about the weather was a question: Why was a nine-year-old riding a tricycle?

After several minutes, she satisfied my curiosity. "He has cerebral palsy. He's just learned to ride the trike. It's good therapy for him."

Cerebral palsy? I had only a vague understanding of what that was. Didn't it cause lack of muscle control? It didn't necessarily mean mental retardation; I remembered reading that.

In the months that followed, we met frequently in the neighborhood as we walked with our sons. We would stop to chat in front of the laundromat or the television repair shop while our children played or slept. Doris talked quietly, telling facts without emotion because she had told them often: "You never expect something like this. It was hard to accept."

I came to see how different mothering was for us. Her son caught a bus to a special school for the handicapped every morning. Her son couldn't speak intelligibly. Her son's achievements came more slowly and with intensive effort.

After we moved from the neighborhood, I never saw Doris or her son again. But they remain strong in my memory. The image I carry is of the boy riding his tricycle in circles on the sidewalk and the mother watching him, unsmiling, eyes narrowed, monitoring his movements.

My husband Jack and I became stateside missionaries in the Pacific Northwest. Occasionally among the congregations in the rural churches we served there would be a handicapped person.

Our hearts ached because we felt inadequate to help these people. We loved them, spent time with them, and gave the best help we knew how, but there were few resources available to us at that time in that location.

After several years, I began to write. As I interviewed people for articles and books, I met more and more disabled people who had stories to tell. Bill was blind; John and Tim were deaf; Judy was in a wheelchair. These people taught me something about what it means to be disabled in a world geared to the able-bodied.

When I traveled I began looking for curb cuts, which allow a person in a wheelchair to move easily from the sidewalk to the street. Were there adequate parking spaces for handicapped people? Were these spaces large enough to accommodate a van with a lift? Could I take a friend in a wheelchair to this restaurant, to that church? Was there an interpreter for the deaf in the worship service?

Their world was melding with mine. I wrote about them more because their needs were becoming important to me.

I wrote about how to relate to a handicapped person—how to create Sunday School programs and other ministries. I wrote curriculum to help able-bodied children relate to handicapped people. But one experience in particular caused me to pray that I'd be able to publish a book on the subject.

That new experience was with Ruth McEwen. Burned over 64 percent of her body as an infant, Ruth was left legally blind and deaf. Surgery and adaptive equipment restored her sight and hearing; additional surgery provided her with limited mobility. Then, through the use of talking books and other helps, Ruth earned four college degrees—including a master's degree in special education and a master's degree in counseling.

Now Ruth is a Rehabilitation and General Counselor—a professional helping handicapped people and their families. Though confined to a wheelchair by the effects of a disease known as lupus, Ruth is active in many organizations that work for the welfare of disabled people. She and my husband and I have become very close friends.

Through our ongoing relationship, I've learned something of how a parent must feel when an offspring is disabled. I want life to be easier for Ruth, to see her experience less pain. Like a parent, I have had to learn that, while I can change some things for her, there are many things I cannot change. But I can share her dreams and goals to help provide the best quality of life possible for other disabled sons and daughters.

One way I've been able to do that is to write this book. It contains the kind of information Jack and I would like to have had years ago while we were leading churches.

So, you see, this book is an answer to prayer. The research I've been doing for years, the tutoring I've received from persons who are disabled, the time I've spent with specialists in the field, and my study of organizations devoted to caring for disabled people, have all been part of God's training.

I pray that once you walk through the lives of the families of handicapped children, once you sense the parents' quiet desperation and their feelings of isolation from the rest of society, you'll want to move alongside them and become involved in their support.

That's one thing these families need—someone who is informed about their particular problems, and who is also willing to help them through the crises they face.

The other thing they need is the love, understanding, and help of the Christian family—the Body of Christ. These families need to experience this supernatural, spiritual bond in practical ways. As Patty McGill Smith, mother of a mentally handicapped, epileptic daughter, puts it, "Pain divided is not nearly so hard to bear as is pain in isolation."

CHAPTER ONE

FAMILIES, FACTS, AND FEELINGS

IT'S A SCENE MOST COUPLES PRAY THEY'LL NEVER HAVE TO play out. At first, everyone is as excited as anticipated. The long-awaited labor pains begin, and husband and wife race to the hospital. He stands by her side in the birthing room while she pants and pushes as she's learned. One final push and there arrives the culmination of months of waiting and planning: *Their baby is here.*

But instead of giving the infant to the mother, medical personnel knot around the newborn in a corner of the delivery room, exchanging sober glances. An incubator is pushed in and the baby is taken away. Exhilaration turns to panic. *Something's wrong with my baby!*

Or the scene may be a couple's living room. Vainly the parents try one more time to get their ten-month-old to sit up. But he flops over like a Raggedy Ann doll. Silently they exchange glances, a sinking feeling in their stomachs. *Something's wrong with our baby.* They consult a physician and hear a dreaded diagnosis.

For some parents, the scene is a crowded emergency room. Frantic, they rush through the door. They've just been told that the bus in which their seven-year-old was riding skidded on an icy road and crashed over an embankment. After an unbearable wait, a physician finally appears. "The injuries are very serious. It involves the spinal cord . . ." *Something awful has happened to our child.*

In each scenario distraught parents, sick with fear, head next for the telephone. Whom will they call? The family physician, if he's not already present. Immediate family members. The prayer chain, if their church has one. Their closest friends. And, of course, their pastor. He's one of the primary people they depend on to provide strength and wisdom in crisis.

Though pastors are often among the first people called upon to help in a crisis, this book is intended to be a resource for any

Christian who is concerned about or involved with families who have handicapped children. It's designed to help not only during the immediate crisis—when the disability is discovered—but also over the long haul as the family adjusts to and lives with a handicapped child.

"When we discovered that our baby had a disability, we got in touch with the pastor. He came right away," Caroline recalls. "He was wonderfully understanding and loving. He prayed with us and tried to comfort us and even cried with us. But in the weeks and months that followed, he admitted that he felt helpless because he wasn't experienced in situations like ours and didn't know what more to do."

Parents don't expect a helper to have all the answers. It's the presence of a caring, ministering person that is needed. "When it happened, all I wanted was someone to listen and let me say everything that I was thinking and feeling," one mother says.

Another reflects, "I needed more than to have the minister come in, ask, 'How are things going?', offer a prayer, and leave." She wishes he'd taken time to find out about her child's condition so that she could talk with him about it.

The Statistics

You, the caring, ministering person, may not have a family with a handicapped child in your congregation now. But since, according to current March of Dimes statistics, almost one-tenth of all children are handicapped in some way, chances are that you will sooner or later.

Handicapped people used to be kept sequestered; now they are being "mainstreamed" into society. That makes it even more likely that a mentally impaired baby will be part of your church nursery, a blind child part of your Sunday School class, or a paralyzed teenager part of your youth group.

But aren't fewer babies born with birth defects these days? Think of the advances in medical science in recent years. Hasn't that made a difference?

Unfortunately, the statistics have not changed. According to the March of Dimes, three in every 100 babies are born with a major birth defect—the same number recorded 20 years ago. One reason is that research in many disorders is still in its infancy. And while some conditions receive a lot of attention, funding, and scientific study, others do not.

One breakthrough that has effectively reduced disabilities is the rubella (German measles) vaccine. Since that development, significant advances have been made in eliminating congenital birth defects that occurred if the mother contracted rubella during her first trimester (three months) of pregnancy. Most rubella-related defects are permanent—conditions such as hearing or visual impairment, heart defects, even behavioral disorders. Perhaps we will see similar progress in other areas. If current educational campaigns concerning drug and alcohol abuse are successful, we might also see a decline in defects caused by these substances.

But there are limits to the progress we can expect in the near future. Even supertechnology such as genetic transplanting, which may hold exciting long-range possibilities, cannot help now. Writing in a 1987 issue of *Newsweek* magazine about the faulty gene that produces birth malformations, Jerry Adler states, "Medical science in all its ingenuity cannot grow a fingernail, let alone a heart. And it has little hope, therefore, of knowing how the process can go wrong."[1]

Some malformations can be detected before birth through tests like amniocentesis. But the only solution for prospective parents who find out their baby has a deformity such as Down's syndrome is to have an abortion—an answer many people, especially Christians, find unacceptable.

D. Gareth Jones, Head of the Department of Anatomy and Human Biology of an Australian university, states that genetic abnormalities are one of the prime reasons cited in defense of therapeutic abortions—abnormalities such as Down's syndrome, hemophilia, disorders resulting from German measles. In the *Journal of the Christian Medical Society* (Vol. 14, No. 1, p.7), Jones writes that some parents may abort a malformed fetus, hoping for a healthy child in the future. He regards this as a step toward making human persons interchangeable. Pointing out that genetic defects are one result of the fall of man, he states, "In general, helping the handicapped, not taking their life in advance, is the way to improve the quality of human life."

Not all congenital defects are detected at birth. In spite of new technology, some problems, such as deafness, may not be discovered until the child is older. In such cases, parents may intuitively know something is wrong with their child; some report an agonizingly long trek to physicians to determine the problem. "My doctor told me I worried too much, that I should just give the baby time. But I finally found one who listened to me and confirmed my suspicions," one parent recalled.

Statistics on birth defects do not include children who develop handicaps after birth as the result of illness or injury. One such illness is encephalitis, an inflammation of the brain which may lead to a variety of physical handicaps.

Other problems may develop during childhood without warning. That's the way it happened for one couple whose two sons developed seizure disorders. Accidents disable still other children, such as Greg, whose story is told in Chapter 2.

What the Words Mean

Our society needs words to describe persons who have physical, mental, of other defective conditions. One of the words used often is *handicapped*, meaning possessing something that hampers a person, something that is a hindrance. Another word is *disabled*, to make unable. Here are two common words that have negative meanings: *invalid* and *cripple*. These words have a pejorative connotation and should be avoided.[2]

The terms we choose are definitely important, for words often become labels. If a girl keeps hearing herself described as *disabled*, she will likely begin to think of herself in terms of her defective condition. It's much more helpful to describe her as "Lisa, a girl with a disability," or "Shari, a girl with a handicap." That way, we define the individual as *a person first* and as disabled second. Instead of conjuring archaic images of inability and dependency in the minds of children and families, we are describing a person—one who has abilities as well as limitations.

Families in Crisis Need Help

To discover that one is the parent of a handicapped child is only the first step on a journey into the unknown. Parents who are suddenly told that their child has cerebral palsy or Down's syndrome or some other condition may know little about the disease or the effects it could have. Often it's hard for families to get accurate information; they may be so emotionally frayed that they can't decide where to begin. And their physician may not have provided the foundation they need.

The Christian helper is a likely person to enable them to get started. That helper, as was mentioned earlier, may be the pastor or lay person who has become intimately involved with the family because he or she has been calling on them or has been summoned in the crisis. Or it may be a Sunday School teacher or youth worker. In some cases, the helping person may be a friend or acquaintance who sees that there is a need for someone to come alongside to provide support in practical, ongoing ways.

The helper may not have had experience with this type of situation but senses God's inner urging to be available. Though no formal training is required, the helper should be empathetic and spiritually mature.

Because these families are in a delicate emotional state, it's urgent that the helping person exercise wisdom in what is said and done. For one thing, the helper should take time to become informed about the particular situation; for another, recognize personal limitations.

A good place for the helper to begin is to acquire general information about the disability the child has.

Types of Disabilities

Joyce S. Mitchell, a consultant in education, former school counselor, and author of several books about children with disabilities. In her book, *Taking on the World*, designed to help parents provide the best quality life for their exceptional child, Mitchell describes four types of disabilities which are as follows:

- *Developmental Disability*—A severe chronic disability involving three or more major life functions (e.g., language, mobility, learning, ability to take care of self) which has an onset before age 22 and is likely to continue indefinitely.
- *Learning Disability*—A condition in which a child whose nervous system is slow in maturing experiences disorder with his or her environment. The child lacks the necessary tools to organize what is seen, heard, touched, felt, smelled, and tasted in order to make sense of the environment.
- *Physical Disability*—A physical impairment that lasts for at least six months and interferes with major tasks of daily living such as walking, seeing, hearing, lifting, talking, and going to work or school.
- *Handicap*—This current definition refers to the effect of a barrier or obstacle in the environment that prevents people with disabilities from performing daily tasks. If the barrier can be removed by providing things such as Braille books or an

interpreter for the deaf, "the disabled person is no longer handicapped for that particular activity."[3]

Here are some general categories of disabilities as listed by the National Information Center for Handicapped Children and Youth and based on the Education for All Handicapped Children Act:

- *Deaf*—An impairment severe enough to prevent the child from receiving linguistic information through hearing, with or without amplification.
- *Deaf-blind*—Simultaneous hearing and visual impairment.
- *Hard of hearing*—A hearing impairment that is less severe than deafness.
- *Mentally impaired*—Below average general intellectual functioning, along with deficits in adaptive behavior. This is the most prevalent of all conditions. The Mental Retardation Association reports that there are six million persons who are intellectually retarded in the United States. Unless significant medical progress is made, 100,000 babies each year are likely to be added to that category. *Down's syndrome* (formerly called mongolism; caused by an extra chromosome) is one of the best known causes of mental retardation. There are over 250 causes of this disability already known.
- *Multihandicapped*—A combination of impairments (such as mental retardation and blindness, or deafness and a seizure disorder).
- *Orthopedically impaired*—Physical disabilities involving the skeletal system. These may be congenital, such as missing limbs or spina bifida (failure of some vertebrae in the spinal column to close properly), or they may result from trauma such as burns.
- *Speech impaired*—A communication disorder.
- *Visual handicap*—A visual impairment, with or without correction.
- *Neurological disorders*—Disabling conditions caused by damage to the central nervous system. Some examples of this type of disorder are cerebral palsy and muscular dystrophy. Also to be noted is *paraplegia* (paralysis of the lower half of the body, affecting both legs) which can result from a spinal cord injury. Other possible causes of this paralysis are aneurysms, infection, and trauma. The extent of paralysis depends on the location of the spinal injury. *Quadriplegia* is paralysis of all

extremities, affecting the upper body as well.

- *Other health impairments*—Including autism, a psychological disorder evidenced by an inability to relate to or communicate with others or one's surroundings.
- *Specific learning disabilities*—Such conditions as perceptual handicap, minimal brain dysfunction, dyslexia, and developmental aphasia.

The list of specific disorders is too lengthy to give here, but a glossary of technical terms is provided in the back of this book.

Parents' Reactions to the News

In recent years, it has become increasingly common for couples to knowingly adopt handicapped children. These couples have presumably prepared themselves for the fact that the children are disabled and will require special parenting skills.

Because these parents don't experience the initial shock of birth parents, they are not specifically referred to in this book. But in practical areas of day-to-day life, adoptive parents will need much the same help as parents to whom a disabled child is born. They'll probably have to search just as hard to find the best therapy and other developmental care; they'll likely experience the same discouragement and need the same kind of counsel.

How do parents feel when they are told their baby is blind, or deaf, or has cerebral palsy? How do they react when told that their child is a quadriplegic as a result of a spinal cord injury?

The latter happened to football star Nick Buoniconti, whose 19-year-old son, Mark, was injured playing football. "Complete helplessness" was the way the senior Buoniconti described his feelings as he looked down at his son in a hospital bed. He said he did what any real man would do—he cried.

Author Patty McGill Smith describes her own reaction and the reactions of other parents:

The day my child was diagnosed as having a handicap, I was devastated—and so confused that I recall little else about those first days other than the heartbreak. . . . Another parent described this event as a "black sack" being pulled down over her head, blocking her ability to hear, see, and think in normal ways. Another parent described the trauma as "having a knife stuck" in her heart. Perhaps these experiences seem a bit dramatic, yet it has been my experience that they may not sufficiently describe the many emotions that flood parents' minds and hearts when they receive bad news about their child.[4]

Some parents say they grieved but did not panic. Because they already had a strong faith in God, they say they were able to trust Him when they learned their child had a disability. "I experienced God's grace," the parent of a deaf child says. But even though such parents sense God's strength, they still feel profound sadness. Recalling their initial crises—most of which happened years ago—more than one parent broke down while sharing the events with me.

"Picture this if you will—you are a brand new mother," says Judith Jogis, as quoted in the book, *The Disabled and Their Parents*. "A strange doctor has just been in to your bedside to tell you—brutally and without preliminaries—that your cherished, new little son has a serious birth defect. . . . You can't believe what you've heard. . . . Another doctor has told your husband that it would be better to let the child die. . . Your heart is in your throat all the time; you feel so empty. Where is the promise of all those months?"[5] Mrs. Jogis is the mother of a congenitally handicapped child.

Physician Charlotte E. Thompson describes some of the stages through which these parents are likely to go. First, they experience shock or "the violent impact on the mind or emotions of an unexpected overwhelming event that comes as a blow." Then numbness usually sets in, a response that Dr. Thompson says "is nature's way of giving us time to withdraw and develop our individual coping mechanisms."[6]

Husband and wife may grieve differently. An individual's emotional responses do not fit a set pattern or occur within a set time frame.

Grieving parents usually feel guilty. They wonder if they might have done more to prevent their child's condition. "Maybe if I had eaten better when I was pregnant or quit work earlier," a mother will say. One mother feared she hadn't paid close enough attention to her son's behavior in the weeks before he began having seizures. Another feared she and her husband hadn't acted quickly enough at the onset of the illness that left her son with a severe handicap. "Maybe if we'd done things differently . . ."

Anger is a common emotion. It may be self-directed, directed toward another family member, the handicapped child whom they then reject, or toward the physician, accusing him or her of incompetence. One parent said, "I was very angry toward the friend who let my daughter drive when she didn't have a license. If they'd acted more responsibly, the accident that disabled her wouldn't have happened.''

You may also encounter parents who passed through the initial crisis years before, but who still have not explored their true feelings or worked through them. ''It takes great maturity to accept a handicap in a child, to learn to cope with it and to continue as a loving, giving person,'' Thompson adds.[7]

Parents aren't the only ones who feel strong emotions. If the child is older at the onset of the disabling condition, he or she will feel them, too. So will siblings, and the extended family—including grandparents. ''My mother was furious with the doctor and wanted to sue,'' said one father whose son became disabled after an acute illness.

Difficult Decisions

During the initial crisis, parents will probably have to make difficult decisions—even as they feel very confused by all that is happening. *Do we need another medical opinion? How hard should we fight to save our child's life? What options for treatment are available? Can we cope with this child's care on a long-term basis? What do we tell family and friends? How are we going to pay for all this?*

One of the most important decisions parents will make is whether or not to care for their child themselves. Several decades ago, institutionalization was common; today experts agree that most disabled children thrive better in a healthy home environment. More and more families are rearing their handicapped children themselves, though it is not always possible to do so. Some parents I talked with never considered foster care or institutionalization for their disabled children—but realized that at some point it may become their only realistic alternative.

Effects on the Family

The tension and extra care involved with parenting a disabled child can severely strain a marriage. Some counselors state that the divorce rate for couples with a chronically handicapped child may be as high as 90 percent.

This alarming statistic should be of special concern to Christians who wish to minister to these families. These families' need for loving support does not stop just because they may appear to have adjusted to the situation; they will need caring people involved in their lives for a long time because of the stress and fatigue which often accompany this special type of parenting.

The single parent of a handicapped child faces the most difficult circumstance of all. Often the mother has custody of the children, and must work to provide for the family. If she has chosen to care for the child at home, she'll need a specially trained baby-sitter—which may be expensive and hard to find. The extra work load the parent must carry, combined with the stress, will sap her energy and eat up time she might have had for herself.

Family members have to deal with the fact that some relatives and friends may have trouble accepting the handicapped child. They must also deal with well-meaning but thoughtless remarks like, "Your situation makes me feel lucky."

Then there are those who, meaning to reassure, say, "Remember that all things work together for good." One parent, to whom that verse was quoted, recalls, "I *knew* that, but I didn't want to *hear* it then."

Perhaps most hurtful are callous statements, sometimes made even by "experts": "Put him in an institution and forget him. He'll always be a vegetable."

Needed: Spiritual Strength

How can families of handicapped children hope to cope? Their needs are many, but one vital ingredient is a strong foundation of faith.

James McAlister, writing in *Moody Monthly* about his own experiences, said his wife Mary was more prepared to adjust to the birth of their blind, profoundly retarded daughter Jenny because Mary had been studying the Bible intensely and he had not. He describes himself as having been a nominal Christian when Jenny was born.

At first, McAlister avoided his daughter and left his wife to care for her. Not until Jenny was hospitalized at two months of age was Mary able to help him understand his actions. After that experience, he opened up to his daughter and became a real father to her.

As with other parents of disabled children, the McAlisters found their love for their handicapped child taking on an extra dimension. It was hard for them to place her in a total care facility, even though they knew the move was best for Jenny. Since making that decision, they've moved closer to the facility so that they can see her every day.

Even though Jenny cannot chew, has no muscle control, and can't speak, she still is a person who communicates and shows distinct preferences. Her father says she likes soft music and delights in being touched. He also believes there is the possibility that, even though her intellectual understanding is extremely limited, her spirit is sensitive and responsive. "If that's true, it would appear she is aware of things that only can be revealed by God's Spirit. . . . (I Corinthians 2:10-13)."[8]

We *know* that these children are important to God. Jesus said that when we care for those generally considered to be "the least" of His brothers, it is as though we are actually caring for Him.

What better motivation could we have to come alongside the families of handicapped children?

The parents whom we are called to help have been knocked flat by one of life's most difficult blows—the trauma of accepting and raising a handicapped child. The family is emotionally overwhelmed, distraught, and confused—possibly with no idea where to turn for help. Since the occurrence of these unfortunate circumstances is not decreasing, the likelihood of having such a family in your church is significant.

As we have seen, these families desperately need a mature, caring Christian to come alongside as a helper—someone like you, who is empathetic, willing to grieve with them, willing to learn about handicaps and how to locate experts to help them, and willing to be available in the event of future crises.

The privilege of being such a helper can be deeply satisfying.

Chapter Two

Case Studies

THE BEST WAY TO UNDERSTAND WHAT IT'S LIKE TO PARENT A handicapped child (unless you have one of your own) is to experience it vicariously through the words of another. The following families were willing to relive the past—painful as it was—so that you could do that. They have spoken openly and honestly, describing their thoughts and feelings, what was helpful in their situations, and what was not. Except for the case of Karlee, Jerry, and Greg, names of the individuals have been changed to protect their identities.

A Disabling Seizure Disorder

Words can't describe how Bruce and Denise felt when their four-year-old daughter, Heidi, suddenly began having seizures that rendered her unconscious in October, 1986. The frequency of the seizures kept increasing. ''Then Heidi also started having ones that threw her out of her chair onto the floor,'' recalls her mother.

The couple took Heidi to a doctor right away, but at first had a hard time convincing him that something was wrong. ''Finally, we had to demand he do a brain scan. We prayed that if she was going to have a seizure, she'd have it when she was having the scan so they'd see it.'' And that's just what happened.

Their daughter was diagnosed as having a seizure disorder (also called epilepsy), but the physicians could not determine the cause of the problem. A pediatric neurologist took over the case and began treating Heidi with medication.

Denise says, ''I wanted to think the doctors could fix [her problem]. One of the greatest revelations of all time was to face the fact that the knowledge doctors have is limited. They are not God.'' Numerous medications are available for seizure disorders, but finding the right one was a matter of trial and error. The next year was a nightmare for Heidi's family as she was first on one medication and then another. Each medication had its own set of side effects—from possible damage to internal organs to soreness and sponginess of mouth and gums.

While Heidi was on one combination of medications, her grand mal seizures became less frequent and, for about two months, stopped completely. But during that time, she began to have as many as 20 unusual seizures daily; her head would drop and her arms would go straight up. If this type of seizure occurred when she was eating, she'd smash her head in her plate of food.

At times Bruce and Denise would have to restrain her so that she could sit up and eat; when things were really difficult, Heidi had to be fed. Petit mal seizures—a type usually of short duration, in which the victim appears to be staring into space—were frequent during this time, too. The physician had a difficult time telling the couple that Heidi's seizure disorder might never go away. Hearing that news was even harder for the couple to take. Heidi was confused by what was happening to her; Bruce and Denise tried to explain it to her by saying that her body wasn't "minding" her.

At this writing Heidi's brother Steve, a year older than Heidi, appears to be trying "to act like an adult" regarding his sister's disability. He never talks about how it affects him, and he tries very hard to help around the house. "Every once in a while, though, he'll have a tantrum and throw himself to the floor," Denise says. "We realize now that when he does that he's trying to tell us he's hurting. Then his dad will play ball with him or he and I will do something together." Bruce and Denise are trying to lower their expectations for Steve as a helper.

Because of the severity of Heidi's seizure disorder, she seems like a different child. Formerly toilet trained, she now has no bladder or bowel control. Some of the medications make her extremely irritable and hyperactive. Her personality has changed; her emotions are affected. "Often she cries uncontrollably at night, even screaming. She may have a seizure and her arm hits the wall and wakes her up," explained Denise.

Much of Heidi's care falls on Denise. Bruce, who graduated from nursing school about the time their daughter's disability began, works nights. When he comes home from work, Denise tries to get a little sleep and then takes over again.

Because she's with Heidi all day long, Denise admits she gets overprotective in the hope of preventing seizures. "I want to keep her on my lap all the time. Bruce is a good balance. He lets her do more things so she can still live like a child.''

Lately, the couple has been extremely depressed—sometimes even angry at God, especially when Heidi hurts herself during a seizure. Though they know God is good, He doesn't seem to them to be acting out of love in this situation. This uncertainty about God is reinforced when other people, who can't see how He could allow such a thing to happen, find it easier to blame the parents. ''It is hard,'' Denise says, ''not to ask ourselves if we've done something to bring Heidi's problem about. We wish we could cope all the time instead of blowing up over little things. When you do,'' she says, ''you start hating yourself.''

People at the church where they worship have been sympathetic and helpful, even though the couple had been attending there only a few months at the onset of Heidi's disability. But gradually people's involvement with the family has decreased. Denise says she knows that's natural because people have their own lives. Bruce and Denise have also had to accept the fact that some people can't emotionally handle being around Heidi because of her seizures. These people feel helpless, inexperienced, and fearful.

Their pastor has been very understanding, but Bruce and Denise had to go outside the church for additional help. They needed direction to resources specific to their situation—for example, qualified people to provide respite care, which is care provided by others in order to allow the primary care giver time to rest and relax; ways to get financial aid; and support groups in their area.

''We are learning to be more honest and not say we're fine when we're not,'' Denise says.

It's important for them to know that God doesn't condemn them when they're depressed and angry, but that He understands. Especially helpful have been assurances from Scripture that suffering is part of living in this world.

''There's more in the Bible about suffering than prosperity,'' Denise observes. ''We know God's not saying, 'How can I make life miserable for that child?' He weeps with us. We have a God who has suffered for us and is helping us bear our suffering now.''

Both parents know how important it is to have time for themselves and to be alone together. But that's not always easy to do. One friend baby-sits and helps with housework; Denise also located a neighborhood woman, experienced in caring for handicapped children, who takes care of Heidi from time to time.

When the couple does get out for an evening together, they find the time consumed with talking about their problems. One big problem is finances. When Heidi began having seizures, Denise quit her job to stay home, in spite of the fact that they had previous medical bills to pay. Because Heidi's disability was a preexisting condition, Bruce's new medical insurance wouldn't cover her care. At this time, bills for Heidi's medications alone total $200 a month. They're inquiring to see whether they can get Medicaid that would pay for certain essentials.

They don't have trouble explaining Heidi's disability to children. "Our biggest problem is with adults," Denise says. Heidi wears a helmet to protect her head, but often her face is bruised from falling. She has an ongoing bump on her forehead and has split her lip frequently. Once her entire face was swollen from smashing down on it. A face guard is going to be added to her helmet for further protection.

"Some people think Heidi's abused and ask what's wrong with her, or they'll tell me I need to take her to a doctor. Some have even asked what we've done to our child. I try to explain that she has seizures; but some people don't believe me; others don't understand about seizures. I rarely take her out anymore because people get so upset."

When the family is at church, people become concerned when Bruce and Denise allow Heidi to play outside on the grass. They're afraid she'll get hurt. Bruce and Denise say it can be hard to do what they feel is right for Heidi when it means some people might misunderstand.

Family life was complicated even more by the fact that Denise was two months pregnant when Heidi's seizures began. Denise gave birth to their third child in the summer of 1987; her responsibilities escalated further. "I find myself shaking all the time," Denise says. "I pray, 'God, if You're going to bring help, please do it now.' "

More recently, the family moved to another state to be near a hospital that specializes in brain surgery on people with seizure disorders. This surgery has been considered for Heidi, since ongoing seizures that cannot be controlled by medication can cause brain damage. At this writing, Heidi is being tested to see whether she's a candidate for this procedure.

A Child with Down's Syndrome

Paula was 39 when Jennie was born. She and her husband, Jeff, hadn't worried that Paula's age might increase the likelihood that their child would have a birth defect. Their first child, 11-month-old Miriam, was healthy; they didn't expect this new baby to be any different.

When the doctor entered Paula's room shortly after delivery with the news that Jennie was mongoloid—a term used in the past for Down's syndrome—Paula was stunned. "He didn't give me much information except to say that if such a child were severely handicapped, he or she would be institutionalized," Paula recalls.

Paula lay in her hospital bed numb with shock. "I wished the doctor had waited until Jeff was present so he could have told us together," she says. Instead, he told them at different times. At first Paula didn't care whether the baby lived or died because she wasn't sure she could handle the situation. When Jeff found out, he was very distressed because he thought Jennie's disability meant she would not live long.

Later that day, a nurse who was a Christian came into Paula's room and asked whether she could pray with her. Paula eagerly consented. Afterward, that nurse stayed and talked with her for a long time.

She told Paula that Jennie's condition was now called Down's syndrome. The nurse cited characteristics of this condition: slanting eyes with folds of skin at the inner corners; a flat bridge of the nose; short neck; and a small head and mouth. But most encouragingly, the nurse told Paula she was not in favor of institutionalizing Jennie.

"I knew this meant Jennie would be mentally retarded, but the nurse also explained that these children lack muscle tone and need therapy to increase that area."

After the nurse left the room, Paula sobbed into her pillow. "One thing I did do was to pray, 'Lord, if I'm going to have to care for a handicapped child, please may it be a physically healthy one.' At that time I didn't know these babies often have bad hearts that require surgery. But Jennie's heart is healthy and her physical condition has always been excellent."

Paula didn't want to hold Jennie at first. But her defenses fell when she was encouraged to go to the nursery window to look at her baby. "She looked so cute and sweet—just like the others."

Sensitively but persistently, the nurse urged her to take Jennie in her arms. "Once I held her, I began to have mixed feelings," Paula recalls. "I thought maybe the diagnosis was a mistake. I could see a few signs of Down's syndrome that had been described to me, but unless someone knew what to look for, they wouldn't be noticed."

Paula and Jeff took Jennie home, but felt terribly inadequate as parents. A month later, the baby had to be hospitalized because she was losing weight. The parents assumed they wouldn't be bringing her home again—that she'd stay in the hospital until she died.

After visiting Jennie on Thanksgiving Day, as she and Jeff got back into their car, Paula thought, *I don't want my baby to die!* That was a dramatic turning point for her as Jennie's mother. A change in formula enabled Jennie to gain weight, and soon she was released from the hospital.

Because the parents didn't know where to turn for help and support, they struggled on their own to learn to care for a handicapped child. At the same time they were dealing with feelings of grief and inadequacy.

Some couples can depend on their parents for help, but Paula's mother and father were dead. Jeff's parents were friendly, but didn't express their feelings. As a result Paula and Jeff felt lonely, knowing few people who could listen to them with understanding.

From the beginning, Jeff and Paula didn't seriously consider institutionalizing their baby, even though the extent of her retardation was unknown. They were told that the state institution would not accept a child under five years of age. The only other institutional care available was a private facility which they could not afford. Foster homes were available for children whose parents could not or would not care for them; but even though Paula and Jeff had no confidence in their ability to be adequate parents for Jennie, they figured they could do as good a job as foster parents could.

After several inquiries, Paula located a physical therapy program at a state university in a nearby town. She enrolled Jennie when the girl was about a month old. The program was designed to teach Down's syndrome babies skills others learn on their own—such as rolling over, reaching for things, picking things up, stacking blocks, etc. Each new skill required constant repetition at home to assure that Jennie would remember it.

This repetitive therapy was done primarily by Paula. Now 40 years of age and without the energy of younger mothers in the program, Paula was often frayed by the stress of regularly transporting Jennie to the university with her sister in tow.

One summer she took Jennie to patterning therapy as well. But when she tried to resume this program the next summer, it proved too much for Paula to handle. "I fell apart and had to quit," she recalls. There were times when she wept from exhaustion and prayed for help in the work with Jennie. All the while she was trying to give attention to Miriam as well.

Paula was encouraged as Jennie made small signs of progress. "We were so excited when she finally took her first step. That had been an exciting time for us with Miriam, but it was much more so with Jennie. It had taken so much work to get her that far. I'd lean her against the sofa and put beads on the floor, just out of her reach, trying to entice her to get them. It was physically and emotionally exhausting, especially because all this time Miriam was demanding attention as well. When Jennie was awake, Miriam was, too.

It seemed to Paula that at every moment she was either programming or feeding Jennie; Down's syndrome babies tend to eat more slowly than other babies do. Every bit of programming had to be written so that the people at the therapy center could go over it. This task made additional demands on her time.

Because of this rigorous schedule, Paula got little time away from the children. Jeff helped when he got home from work, but his time with Jennie was limited.

Because she often was close to exhaustion, Paula depended strongly on prayer and strengthening from Scripture to carry her through. She joined a support group, but dropped out when Jennie got older.

Jennie's physical therapy program ended when she was two and a half because, at age three, she was scheduled to enter the school's program for handicapped children. This publicly funded education proved generally satisfactory.

From the beginning, Jeff and Paula took Jennie with them to church and left her in the nursery. Because handicapped children often don't get much exposure to others, they felt that was especially important. "I made it a point to have people hold her. When she started clinging to me in church, I'd leave her with a friend and walk away to visit with others. It was for her own good—and mine, too."

With no special educational facilities in Sunday School, Jennie has had to pick up what she can from teachers who take special interest in her. Some pastors have made extra efforts to establish a close friendship with her; she was especially sad when one of them moved to another community.

Now, at age 12, Jennie can read simple books. She does household chores such as vacuuming and setting the table—skills she's learned through repetition. She loves to visit with people, but it takes patience and experience for most people to understand her.

As Jennie enters adolescence with a 12-year-old's body and a five-year-old's mind, Paula and Jeff say they need help. "How do you explain menstruation to a mentally retarded child?" Paula asks. Jennie wants to be part of the teenage crowd at church, but she isn't and feels left out. The couple is considering talking to their pastor about it.

Her parents have tried to explain the Gospel to Jennie. "She has the understanding of a five-year-old, and I tell myself that a five-year-old can understand it. But it may take someone besides me to make it clear to her."

No one knows yet the extent of Jennie's educability or whether she'll be able to contribute significantly to her own care and support. Consequently, the couple's thoughts about the future are unsettled. "We've told Miriam that we'll never make her promise to take care of her sister, only to keep in touch with her."

The future will have to wait. Right now, dealing with the present seems all this family can handle.

A Case of Severe Brain Damage

When Robin was three months old, her heart stopped. Even though eight years have passed since that night, her mother, Elaine, still breaks down when she recalls the scene. "Glen was holding her. One minute she was fine and the next she was unconscious. We didn't know what was wrong with her. We ran with her to the car and raced to the hospital, attempting to give her CPR [cardio-pulmonary resuscitation, a first-aid measure to revive a person who is not breathing and has no pulse] on the way.''

Until that day, as far as her parents knew, Robin was a normal, healthy baby. But she'd been losing weight and her pulse rate had been fast since birth. So, earlier that day, they had taken her to the doctor for her checkup. He ordered a chest X-ray; that's when they discovered that Robin had an enlarged heart.

Glen and Elaine know now that it would have been better to call an ambulance when Robin's heart stopped. But the doctors in the emergency room were able to revive her; they rushed her the same night by ambulance to a children's hospital in a nearby city. This was the same hospital where, during her checkup, she'd been scheduled for a heart catheterization the next day. How long Robin's heart had been stopped, no one knows. But it was long enough to cause severe brain damage.

A month later, Robin's condition was stable enough for her to leave the hospital. ''Take her home,'' doctors told the couple, ''and give her lots of love. That's what she needs most—to feel loved and secure.'' Almost as an afterthought, Elaine recalls, the doctors told them that Robin was blind.

Back home, Glen and Elaine watched helplessly as Robin lay in her crib, rigid and completely unresponsive, sucking on a pacifier. She bore little resemblance to the happy, healthy baby she'd been a month before.

Robin was their firstborn, so Glen and Elaine were inexperienced at parenting. But even a houseful of normal children couldn't have prepared them for what they faced.

The grief they felt was overwhelming. They felt guilty, too. *If we'd done things differently, wouldn't Robin be different now?*

Glen was angry at the doctors for not discovering Robin's heart condition sooner. Elaine thinks perhaps his feelings were more intense because he had been holding Robin when her heart stopped.

''I was hurting very badly myself,'' reflected Elaine. ''Fortunately, though, years before, I had determined that God knew me. He knew everything that was going to happen. So, whatever did happen was right for me.'' Although she didn't ask ''Why me?'' the way many parents do, she did mourn the healthy child she'd lost, and she agonized for the one Robin had become.

Since Glen and Elaine had to get on with life and attempt to tackle the monumental task of dealing with a severely handicapped child, they tried to push their feelings into the background. Sometimes the anguish of seeing Robin's motionless form seemed more than they could bear. They tried to talk to each other about how they felt, but neither had counseling to know how to deal with their intense emotions.

"We had to do something to at least make her comfortable," Elaine says. Doctors had not given the couple names of people to contact as resources, nor any procedures to follow with Robin. "I remember feeling so lost that first year, so frustrated, because I didn't know where to turn. Not only that, we had no idea what her prognosis was, how much improvement we could expect her to make. At first her heart was a concern, too. Thankfully, though, that has been overcome nicely. Her last tests showed that her heart is very healthy. We're so glad to be finished with that chapter."

Because they supposed Robin was deaf as well as blind, they called the state school for the deaf for advice. This assumption later proved wrong, but when they described Robin's medical history—that she no longer had the use of her limbs and was unable to hold up her head—one of the school's personnel said it sounded as though she had cerebral palsy resulting from the brain damage. That was the first time Glen and Elaine heard a term or label used referring to their child. That also proved to be the correct diagnosis.

The same staff member from the school for the deaf told them that Robin needed physical therapy. With that meager information to go on, Elaine called around her area until she located a physical therapist who worked with cases like Robin's.

In the beginning, the therapist came to Glen's and Elaine's home and showed them how to relax Robin's muscles and stretch them. It was important to keep her muscles loose and help her achieve whatever use of her hands she could. Since Robin had no sense of balance, they worked on that area as well.

Because Glen was busy with his job, Elaine performed most of the physical therapy. She worked daily with Robin, even learning to carry her in a way that would stretch Robin's muscles and encourage the child to hold up her head.

Especially because Robin was blind, Elaine was instructed to talk to her continually in order to stimulate her learning process.

But shortly after her first birthday, tests showed unmistakably that her sight had returned. Theories vary as to why this happened. Some believe new brain cells took over ones damaged when Robin's heart stopped; others feel that the shock to her brain simply wore off sufficiently so that her vision was restored. Glen and Elaine were ecstatic, especially since progress in other areas was very, very slow. Robin still had no control of her arms and legs and still couldn't walk.

From the beginning, people were mostly sympathetic. "We were anxious to talk about [Robin] and appreciated people who asked questions," Elaine recalls. They also appreciated friends who sat with Robin from time to time so Elaine could get out. "I knew I had to have a separate life; I couldn't center it around one child."

But some friends backed away, perhaps because they didn't know how to deal with what had happened. Glen and Elaine were especially hurt when one couple who had been very close became distant and aloof. "There was a time when I didn't have a single close friend and felt desperately lonely," she remembers. She prayed about it, and says that ever since she's had a series of people come into her life. As in most such families, social contact was less of a problem for Glen because he left the home every day to maintain his business.

Like parents of most other disabled children, Glen and Elaine realized that a church usually is not set up to provide special Christian education classes for children like Robin. Still, one of the pastors at their church took it upon himself to see that Robin is taken downstairs every Sunday for children's church so that Elaine can teach a class without being concerned about Robin.

When people take a special interest in Robin, Glen and Elaine are grateful. "For several years, one little girl assigned herself to Robin; when this girl moved on to another class, another took over," Elaine said. They also are grateful when a teacher notices things that especially interest Robin, such as music, and uses that to involve her in the class. "Sometimes, a child will put a crayon in her hand and help her color." Elaine says they probably should let people in the Christian education department know more about how Robin communicates and how to work with her. She feels they have not been as assertive as they need to be in this regard.

Robin had begun attending school part time when she was

two. At four, she was still going to school a few hours a day when Glen's and Elaine's second child, Maryann, was born. By herself, Elaine took care of both children all that summer. "I remember feeding them at the same time, using both hands. Fortunately, Maryann was a contented baby and easy to care for."

Like Robin, most children in her special education class are in wheelchairs and unable to talk; they can't socialize with each other. But Robin is learning to communicate visually—by eye pointing. Here is an example of how this system works: The teacher holds up two different number cards—a three and an eight, for example. The teacher asks which number is the eight, and Robin answers by focusing her eyes on the correct card. Glen's and Elaine's biggest frustration is trying to find a more extensive system of communication that will work for Robin.

The constant regimen and the necessity of devoting so much time and energy to Robin puts stress on marriage and family life for this couple. It's hardest when Glen has to be away for the weekend and Elaine is left alone with the children. She tries hard not to expect too much from Maryann. "It can be a bitter trial for a sibling," Elaine says. So far, Maryann hasn't asked many questions about Robin. But Elaine is pregnant again and wonders what will happen when Maryann has to share even more the attention she gets from her parents.

Especially now that she's pregnant, Elaine depends on Glen's help when he gets home from work. He gives Robin her bath, plays with her, and feeds her an evening snack. If she cries during the night—usually because she wants her position changed—he's the one who gets up.

With two children, one of them in a wheelchair, Elaine doesn't take them shopping often. It's easier to wait until she has a sitter. Times when she has taken them, she manages by hoisting Maryann into the shopping cart, pushing it with one hand and pushing Robin's wheelchair with the other.

People stare at Robin. Elaine says, "Sometimes it bothers me more than others. I feel as though, because she's different, we stand out like an oddity. On occasion, someone gushes at us, 'Oh, you poor thing.' I don't appreciate that. We often wind up giving those people a pep talk."

Glen and Elaine have been advised that since Robin has no mobility by now, she'll probably always be in a wheelchair. She may be mildly retarded as well. "We try to set realistic goals for her level of achievement and strive for as normal a homelife as possible."

The couple is painfully aware that they may not be able to care for Robin at home indefinitely. So they try to make the minutes count. They spend time, not just caring for her, but giving her loving attention. "We see this as a lifetime commitment, so we'll care for her as long as we're able to do so."

A Hearing-impaired Child

Jo contracted rubella (German measles) when she was pregnant with her first child. "We were really ignorant, but we knew there was a possibility our baby could be born with a disability. I had assumed that if something was wrong, either there'd be a spontaneous abortion, or it would be correctable through surgery or some kind of treatment."

Sam was small at birth because the disease had stunted the development of the placenta. Because of this Jo and Ralph knew their child had been affected by the rubella but no testing to determine the extent of its effects was done at that time.

It was Jo's mother who first became suspicious that something was wrong with the baby's hearing. The couple had left ten-month-old Sam with her while they went on a weekend trip. When they returned, she told them that she'd had the baby in the yard in a playpen, and when Jo's father came home, he honked the horn, but the baby didn't turn around.

Jo described the incident to their doctor during the next visit. The doctor sat Sam on a table and tapped it. The baby, alert because of strange surroundings, looked all around. The doctor assured Jo, "Give it time. This is your first baby and you're a little nervous."

Still worried, Ralph and Jo kept trying to test their son's hearing at home. "But he was so alert we couldn't sneak up on him. If we opened the door of the room where he was sleeping, he'd be awake very quickly. We thought it was because he heard us or some other noise, but we know now it was the change in air currents that awakened him. He also could feel the wooden floor vibrate. Sometimes, they would manage to sneak in and put a radio turned on full volume next to his ear. He wouldn't even flinch.

Those months were extremely trying. "Deep in our hearts, we

knew,'' Jo says. But then our hopes would soar when Sam seemed to respond to sounds.

''He really did hear that!'' they'd tell each other excitedly. Other times, when they called or clapped out of his line of vision, he would make no response, and hope vanished.

When Sam was 17 months old, the terrible uncertainty ended. Jo's sister had been taking care of Sam while his parents were away. She had four children of her own and knew kids. She was certain something was wrong with her nephew's hearing and told Ralph and Jo that when they returned.

The next day Jo and Sam were again in the doctor's office. ''They used tuning forks on Sam and he didn't respond at all.'' The physician made an appointment with an ear specialist who put Sam in a soundproof room. Different kinds of noises were introduced that got louder and louder, but the baby acted as though he heard none of them.

The couple was advised to take Sam to a children's hospital for evaluation. Again, Sam was put in a soundproof room into which noises were fed. Jo and her mother were in the room with the baby. ''It was the most noise I've ever been subjected to in my life,'' Jo recalls. ''It made my nerves just wild. I wanted desperately to get out of there. But Sam never paid any attention.''

When it was over, the physician told Jo, ''I'm not going to tell you your child doesn't hear. I'm going to tell you he didn't hear today.''

Jo found the doctor's attitude frustrating. Although advised to wait for Sam to mature before undergoing further evaluation, she told the physician, ''We're not going to wait.''

He responded, ''Well, Mother, you just don't believe!''

Another specialist with the reputation of being one of the best in the field tested Sam again. When Sam's eyes dilated at one sound, the physician exclaimed, ''He hears!'' When she repeated the same sound, Sam looked up in response. Jo cried with joy. ''It was the first time I'd ever *seen* him hear anything.''

At 19 months, Sam was fitted with hearing aids. They allowed the boy to hear certain background noises but not voices. That's when Jo and Ralph looked at Sam and admitted to themselves, ''Our son is deaf.''

Jo recalls, ''It was such a sad time for us. But we never thought 'Why us?' We were never resentful. We grieved but not in anger. And eventually we even came to feel we were special to have a special baby. I think that attitude was the result of God's grace operating in our lives."

Like many rubella babies, Sam is multihandicapped. In addition to deafness, he has an area of visual blackout in one eye, but that impairment doesn't interfere with his life.

The John Tracy Clinic in Los Angeles for hearing-impaired children was near where the family lived. They attended classes one night a week for three years. In these classes they received instruction in how to work with their child.

This clinic emphasized lipreading rather than sign language. Jo and Ralph met people whose children had significant success with this program. They expected Sam would be able to read lips well and eventually speak normally. What they didn't know then was that, on the average, only half of the English language is lipreadable. Conditions for lipreading must be exactly right—the other person can't be chewing gum, have an accent, wear a moustache, etc. "And to expect a person who's never heard the human voice to speak normally is too high an expectation," Jo says now.

During those years, Jo talked to Sam continually, repeating the same word over and over since a deaf child has to see it on the speaker's mouth thousands of times before he can lip-read it. "It took him six months to get his first word, which was 'baby.' I'd been talking constantly about things I was doing for his baby brother—feed the *baby,* change the *baby,* bathe the *baby.* Then one day, Sam was helping me bake bread when I heard the baby crying and exclaimed, 'Oh, no, the baby!' Sam jumped off the stool on which he was standing and ran to the baby. That's when it hit me—*he got that word.*"

Sam did learn to lip-read a few more words. But when he was almost four, the family decided to move to another state so he could attend the state school for the deaf. Jo and Ralph were still holding on to the idea that Sam would learn lipreading and speech. Sign language was not being used at school or at home.

Three years later, the school began a total communication program. This involved using written words, sign language, pictures, spoken words—every possible method of teaching language. At the same time, Jo and Ralph began using sign language at home. That's when Sam really began to learn to communicate. Although he doesn't speak and has limited ability to read lips, he uses sign language fluently.

Jo learned early that, as Sam's primary care person, she was the one who was going to have to be his advocate. Although it was extremely time-consuming, it was easier for her than for some parents because Jo is naturally outgoing and energetic. She kept in close contact with his teachers. "I felt like I could have gotten Parent of the Year award for bugging them so much," Jo said. But she wishes she'd known more about Sam's education rights earlier so she could have asked for a speech tutor for him.

One of the most heartbreaking aspects of Sam's disability has been his isolation from his peers. As a day student in a school where most others were residents, Sam was an outsider. And he didn't have many friends in the community where he lived because these children didn't use the same "language" as Sam. "He went through many lonesome times. Summers were very hard. There just wasn't anyone around like him." Jo and Ralph felt helpless at these times.

Sam played with his younger brother, but their communication was limited, although his brother was always Sam's advocate and a big help to him. His brother kept praying that Sam would be able to hear because he wanted so badly to talk to Sam. Jo and Ralph also prayed for healing—if it was God's will. But they also prayed that, if it wasn't, God would supply strength for all of them to deal with Sam's deafness.

"We have never felt that Sam was a burden. Certainly it takes an enormous amount of extra effort to work with a deaf child." Things that hearing children pick up naturally, these children have to be taught.

Discipline is especially important. While Ralph is naturally more of a disciplinarian than Jo, the couple agreed from the outset that they had to be consistent and firm. "If Sam started running across the street and we said 'stop,' he'd better do it every time." Achieving that kind of obedience has tried their patience, especially when Sam realized at about two years of age that, if he didn't want to pay attention, he could just shut his eyes.

Going to church was pretty boring for Sam. Ralph and Jo finally realized that his conduct in church was more than childish misbehavior. "Sam couldn't hear the music or anything that was going on. No wonder he was bored. When he was three years old, he hid under the table in Sunday School. Later on, I asked him why. He said he was scared. All the people were big and he was little. Their mouths were opening and closing and he didn't understand what was going on.'' But when he was seven, a member of the congregation began interpreting the worship service in sign language. That made all the difference.

Jo thinks it's the loneliness that has been the worst part of Sam's disability for him to cope with. ''I think the reason Sam survived is that he had a loving, caring family, and a number of kids at church reached out to him.''

Now graduated from high school, Sam's new dilemma, one that also concerns his parents, is getting an opportunity to prove what he can do in the workplace despite his disability.

''He says he likes being deaf because nobody bothers him. But all the time he's saying that, I wonder if he's wishing that he wasn't.''

A Child Disabled by Trauma

Seventeen-year-old Greg didn't see the locomotive coming as he approached the railroad crossing that summer evening in 1979. Whether the signal lights were working, Karlee and Jerry are not sure. Greg was driving into the sun and could have been blinded by it.

Upon impact, the top of the car was torn off, and Greg was thrown onto the ground nearby. Seeing that Greg was bleeding from the mouth, an uninjured passenger positioned him so he wouldn't choke.

It was about 9:30 p.m. when Karlee and Jerry received the phone call telling them Greg had been in an accident. ''When we got to the emergency room, no one seemed able to tell us anything about Greg's condition,'' the parents recall. ''We were scared sick anyway, and when we were told he'd been hit by a train, we were devastated.''

The couple asked that their family physician be called. As soon as he arrived, this family friend went into the surgery department and returned with a report on their son's condition. Greg had sustained massive head, lung, and kidney injuries. His entire left side was torn up. That evening five specialists worked on him.

One of the people Karlee and Jerry called from the hospital that night was their pastor. ''The main way he helped was by just being there, listening, and letting us come out with whatever feelings we were having. He tried to answer any questions we had. He just let us talk about whatever came to mind, whether it was denial or the idea that, however much Greg recovered, it would be okay.''

Although the couple didn't realize it that night, Greg and his condition would be the center of their existence for years to come. Because Karlee was at the hospital most of the time, she would not have the energy to invest in other family relationships.

From the beginning, Karlee kept praying, ''Dear God, let him live. Let him live!'' She says she just wasn't ready to part with him and didn't ask herself what kind of life he might have as a result of his massive injuries.

Others in the family did ask, however, about the quality of life Greg now might have. They wondered whether he would want to live unless he could have a reasonably full life. For Jerry, there was still another consideration. Himself a victim of multiple sclerosis, he worried how his wife could survive when and if his own condition deteriorated and she had two disabled people to care for.

The first time the couple saw Greg that night, he was completely covered with bandages from head to abdomen. All they could see were his eyes. He was in a coma. Doctors didn't expect him to live.

Karlee, however, was vehement about the circumstances. *Greg had to live!* She insisted the doctors do everything possible to make that happen. ''I was never a very vocal person before, but Greg's accident brought out things in me I didn't know were there,'' she recalls. ''Sometimes I wonder if doctors did more for him than they would have for another patient because they had this woman on their hands who kept pounding at them, 'Don't let him go.' ''

Karlee spent every day at the hospital with Greg and, along with other family members, did everything she knew to try to restore him from his comatose state. But Greg remained unresponsive.

At first, Jerry and Karlee were dazed with shock and numbed with grief. ''Then I became very angry—at the engineer of the train and at people whom I thought might have helped prevent the accident. And I felt guilty, too. Could we have done something differently so that things would not have turned out this way? I often got very depressed. The son we had was gone; now we had a totally different son. No matter how much we wanted to, we couldn't turn back the clock.''

Karlee's brother and sister and their families came a number of times to help. Friends from their small church were supportive. The couple believes that it was talking with their pastor, friends, and family that most helped them work through their feelings.

After a year of hospitalization, therapists succeeded in getting Greg out of the fetal position with his body curved and his arms and legs drawn toward his chest. But he was still in a partial coma and almost totally paralyzed. Doctors told the family that he'd always be a vegetable because of his massive brain injuries. If any changes were going to take place, they'd happen within the next year and a half.

Greg was to be transferred from the hospital to a rehabilitation center. But it would be a week before a bed would be available.

Karlee wanted to bring Greg home for that week. Physicians and family advised against it because of the time and care Greg required. He was paralyzed, being fed through a tube to his stomach, and had no bowel or bladder control. But because Karlee wanted so badly to try it, the family agreed.

She says, ''They did it for me. They knew I had to try it. Besides, there was no place else for him besides a nursing home.''

The evening after Greg came home, he was seated in his wheelchair in the living room with the rest of the family, still unresponsive and in a partial coma. Greg's dad began tossing a soft, sponge rubber ball to Greg—one of the medical staff had used it in the hospital to try to stimulate him to respond. When the ball fell in Greg's lap and rolled on the floor, Jerry kidded Greg good-naturedly. That's when the family saw Greg respond for the first time—he turned up the corners of his mouth in an unmistakable smile. This was a milestone event! Greg gave his family evidence he was coming out of the coma.

After that week, Greg spent eight months in the rehab center. He then seemed to reach a plateau in his progress. He was still being fed by a stomach tube, still with no bladder or bowel control, still paralyzed and unable to talk. The couple was advised to put him in a nursing home or institution.

''But I couldn't stop there,'' Karlee says. So she and Jerry took him home and worked with him day after day. They also took him for physical therapy when a new facility opened up at a local hospital.

Caring for a youth who is handicapped usually requires major changes at home. Adaptive equipment, health-care products—perhaps a respirator—may fill formerly empty spaces. For a child in a wheelchair, a ramp may be necessary if there are steps to be climbed. Fortunately for Karlee and Jerry, their front door only had one step, and they could manipulate Greg's wheelchair over it. Greg did require a hospital bed. Because it was too big to get into a bedroom, it was placed in the living room.

Sometimes wheelchairs won't go through inner doorways, but since their home was quite new, it had been built with the wider doorways newer homes have. Transporting Greg away from home was a problem, however. For quite a while, Karlee transferred him from wheechair to family vehicle herself. Eventually that got to be too difficult so they purchased a van with a wheelchair lift.

After several months they were able to remove Greg's feeding tube. Three and one-half years after his accident, he began to walk. Karlee and Jerry believe he made this progress because he was happy at home and felt secure with his family.

"He still can't talk, but he understands very well. He communicates with gestures and by drawing pictures." Although he understands words, he still isn't able to write them yet.

For a while, Greg was working in a sheltered workshop doing landscaping. As he regained more ability, he started working several hours a day in a bank under a supervised program. Although he still lives at home, Karlee and Jerry believe that the next step may be to help him set up an apartment with another handicapped person where a caretaker would visit daily and provide needed supervision.

"We have a boy who loves life and is full of love—and is the biggest tease in the world," Karlee says. But she doesn't believe her way of handling a situation like Greg's is for everyone. "I think parents should do what they as individuals feel they can and want to do. We do all need to reach for the best quality life-style our handicapped children can have."

"Since I was the one who kept pushing him, I did keep asking myself, 'Am I being foolish? Selfish? Doing this for Greg? Or myself?' "

If Karlee had things to do over, she'd give more time and

attention to her younger son and to her husband. "I'm still dealing with guilt because of that." She believes that the stress of the past years has caused her husband's health to deteriorate more rapidly than it might have.

One thing she still cannot handle is to look at a family picture taken before Greg's accident. "If I do, the old anger rises up in me. But I've learned I simply can't dwell on the past."

When she and Jerry look at Greg, however, they're thankful that his future looks pretty bright.

CHAPTER THREE

QUESTIONS AND ANSWERS

PARENTS OF CHILDREN WITH DISABILITIES ARE OFTEN BOMbarded with questions that whirl in their thoughts. This chapter attempts to address many of those questions in a conversational style. One of the most distressing and frequently asked questions, ''How could a loving God allow this to happen?'' will be extensively covered in Chapter 6.

Our child was born with a disability. How can I get over my fear that I can't cope with this?

It's natural for you to feel overwhelmed at the idea of parenting a handicapped child. It may help to realize that what your child needs most is love—the same thing every child needs. In that respect, your child isn't to be treated differently than any other child. The best antidote for the fear and uncertainty you are experiencing is to educate yourself about your child's disability. As your knowledge increases, so will your confidence. Every time you do something constructive for your child, your feeling of being overwhelmed will subside a little more.

My doctor says my child is a vegetable. I don't want to believe it. What do you think?

No child can ever become a vegetable. No matter how diminished his or her capacity, that child has been created in God's spiritual image and has value. Such terms as ''vegetable'' prejudice parents against children who are unresponsive and unable to communicate. Instead of such inappropriate terms, insist that medical personnel use concrete words to describe your child's disability, not ones that attempt to assess his or her human state. Only time and work will reveal what any child's capabilities are. View your child the way God does, as a person to be loved.

I feel as though I'm on an emotional roller coaster since our child became disabled. How can I control my feelings?

Such feelings are normal for someone who's been through your experiences. While you do want to keep your emotions in check, instead of trying to squelch them, talk openly about them with someone who understands. Some find it helpful to talk to another parent of a handicapped child. If you don't know such a person, contact an organization designed to help parents that is listed in the bibliography in the back of this book. Or you may choose to talk with your pastor or another Christian helper. Simply verbalizing the way you feel is a release—especially feelings that may keep you from accepting your child. Anyone who has weathered crises of their own will assure you they have shared your ups and downs. You are not alone. Jesus Himself experienced extreme negative emotions in the Garden of Gethsemane. He poured them out to His Father and then chose to do what He knew was His Father's will (Matthew 26:36-46; Luke 22:39-46).

My daughter is mentally handicapped. As she gets older, how do we help her accept Jesus Christ as her Savior? How can we know she understands the Gospel?

You will want to talk about the Lord with her on a regular basis, helping her become aware that He is part of your everyday life. Then, when it comes to explaining the Gospel story, she will already be familiar with this important Person in your life.

Explain the Gospel to her simply, slowly, and in small pieces. (Curriculum is available for teaching mentally impaired children; see the Bibliography for suggestions.) Use simple visual aids to explain God as Creator. Repeat stories as much as necessary until she seems to understand. Then introduce a new story about God, building on what has already been learned. Songs appropriate for her mental age can be a helpful way to teach important truths.

You might find the attitude of this mother helpful. Her daughter is 12 but has the mental age of a 5-year-old. She confidently stated, "I know my mentally impaired daughter can become a Christian because the Gospel is so simple." This mother knows she has to wait until her daughter shows she's ready to make a decision to accept Jesus as her Savior. She will wait until her daughter really understands and doesn't simply parrot what she's heard. (These principles are true for all children. The mentally handicapped, though, need more time.)

As you teach your daughter, be aware of her mental age, using words and methods appropriate for that age group.

Here are clues that will indicate your daughter understands what you've been teaching: she will talk about salvation spontaneously, using her own words; she will indicate her desire to please God; spiritual conversations will take place without coaching.

This personal incident showed me (the author) that a mentally impaired youth can have a personal relationship with Christ and give solid evidence of that fact. Once, when my husband and I were visiting a nursing home, we talked with a young man who was mentally handicapped.

"Wait a minute," he said to us. "I want to show you something." He walked to a shelf, took down a Bible, and spoke with conviction. "Know what this is? It's the Word of God. It tells that Jesus is our Savior and will take us to Heaven when we die. That's what's going to happen to me because He's my Savior."

That was one of the most powerful witnesses about the Gospel of Christ I've ever heard.

My wife and I are exhausted from taking care of our severely handicapped daughter. We hardly even converse anymore.

You need to build a support system to help you carry the load. Your circumstances must not let you sacrifice your marriage relationship. God is your primary source of strength, so stay close to Him. Then assess your options. Do you have family or close friends who are at ease with your daughter and can help? What about people in the church? Be honest with the pastor or church leader about your situation. Contact your social worker, physician, physical therapist, or other parents of handicapped children for direction. You need to find respite care so you can get away alone with your wife.

You'll probably have to shift priorities somewhat and learn to live with fingerprints on the walls and clutter in the garage. Use the help God provides to do the most important things, such as spending time relaxing with your spouse or your other children. It's imperative to have rest periods when you can relax with each other and just talk. Don't feel as though you are imposing on others by asking for help. God means for Christians to help one another at times like these.

I thought parents just naturally loved their babies, but I don't feel that way toward my son who has spina bifida. What's wrong with me?

During pregnancy, parents harbor a fantasy image of their child-to-be. Physician Charlotte E. Thompson points out that a mother sees childbearing as fulfillment of herself as a woman; fathers see it as evidence of manhood. Both anticipate a perfect baby and the pleasure of showing off their new offspring. When fantasies aren't fulfilled, we may feel cheated.

Your son has physical malformations that may even be repugnant to you. That doesn't mean you're abnormal, only shocked at this turn of events because you were unprepared to deal with them.

Are you blaming yourself for this disability? Does his condition make you feel inferior? These and other attitudes can prevent you from bonding to your son. Resolving these attitudes removes the barriers and frees you to establish a loving relationship with him. It will help to keep in mind that "love comes from God" (I John 4:7). Ask Him to help you see the wonderful, lovable qualities about your child.

Where can I find the information I need to understand my daughter's condition? Our doctor hasn't explained things so I can understand them, nor has he told me what to do for her.

Ask the attending physician specific questions to which you want answers. Don't worry if they seem elementary. You may want to write these questions in advance so you won't forget any in the nervousness of the moment. If he uses language you don't understand, be sure to ask him to put it in layman's terms.

A large number of informational agencies exist. Call or write ones that apply to your situation. (See suggestions in this bibliography.) Many will send informational literature; some publish newsletters. Obtain recently published books on the subject. Contact your area medical school or a university with special programs in the field for help. Explore these avenues and you'll soon be building up a resource of knowledge. This will help you be able to make informed decisions about your child's care.

Should I accept the doctor's diagnosis or get a second opinion?

There's nothing wrong with asking for a second or third opinion and many parents do that. Besides settling the agony of not knowing what's wrong, it's important to have a correct evaluation as early as possible so your child can begin whatever therapy may be recommended. The earlier this gets started, the more progress your child will have a chance to make.

If you suspect something is wrong but your physician doesn't concur, or if you have evidence to believe your child has been misdiagnosed, take him or her to someone who has been recommended and has good credentials. Often it is wise to seek a diagnosis at a clinic or hospital because there will be physicians with different specialties available. If a child is multihandicapped, making a diagnosis can be complicated. Of course, it's futile to run from doctor to doctor trying to find one who tells you what you want to hear.

Should we keep our handicapped son at home or look for an institution to provide his care? Are there other options?

Many factors are involved in making this decision. Is there someone who can provide the necessary care for this child? Does that person also have to care for other disabled or dependent people such as another handicapped child or an elderly parent? As parents, your own emotional and physical stamina must be considered. So must the severity of the handicap your son has. Does he require a large amount of equipment or therapy, for example? Is your home life relatively stable?

More and more evidence has been shown that the love and acceptance that can be provided in a home environment play a major role in the progress a disabled child makes. The plethora of organizations that exist now to help those with various kinds of disabilities has enabled more parents to care for their children at home.

It is a good idea to talk this over with an informed person not directly involved in the situation. It's essential that both parents make the decision together, that they make it prayerfully, and that most of all, they consider the well-being of the child.

If your son can't be cared for effectively at home, don't allow yourself to be consumed with guilt. If desired, you usually can change your decision at a later time. A child committed to an institution or put in foster care can be brought home; a child taken home can later be institutionalized, put in a special residence, or placed in foster care.

Why can't someone tell me what my child's potential will be?

No expert can foretell the future of a child. So it follows that they can't predict the level of achievement of a disabled child. For one thing, a young child's natural abilities, personality, and characteristics are unknown and undeveloped. That's why parents and others need to provide all the opportunities they can to develop their child's potential.

There are even more reasons why the level of achievement of a handicapped child cannot be spelled out. It's impossible, for example, to accurately test the level of retardation of a Down's syndrome infant. Likewise, the degree of mobility a child with cerebral palsy can achieve is discovered during the therapy process. Periodic evaluations of your child are important and enable new goals for his or her development to be set. Your child may or may not reach all of them, but what's important is to provide the opportunity.

I'm a single parent. How can I possibly handle this situation?

Unquestionably, you'll need lots of help. If you plan on keeping your child at home and you also have to work, you will need someone qualified to care for your child.

All parents need a network of support, but you even more so. Ask God to supply the extra hands you need and someone who can give you emotional support. Be open with people from your church, friends, and family members when they ask "Can I do something?" Perhaps someone will become an adopted grandparent to your child.

Probably one of your most urgent, ongoing needs is financial. Raising any child takes money; caring for and rearing a child with a disability is even more expensive. If you are divorced and have been awarded child support, are the payments being made consistently? If not, you may have to ask the court to intervene.

You may have hospitalization that covers the majority of expenses, but if you don't, investigate some alternatives to help cover medical care, adaptive equipment, etc. (See suggestions in Chapter 7.)

Your church may be able to help with things you'd normally have to spend money for, such as baby-sitting. When people from the church ask how they can help, let them know your real needs—special food for the baby, medical supplies, gas money to drive to therapy, etc.

Most of all, learn to count on God as a real, present Father to yourself and your children. Your great financial need can become an opportunity to learn to trust Him to provide however He will. It's important not to write scenarios in your mind in which *you* decide how He will meet your financial need. Otherwise, if God doesn't act out your script, you may become angry at Him and disillusioned with Christians through whom you expected Him to provide.

When you prioritize your needs, put time for yourself near the top. Ask members of your Bible study, a prayer partner, or close friend to help you find creative ways to do so. Otherwise, the strain of working day and night will exhaust you and make you less able to parent the way you want to.

You'll need someone to talk to regularly about your frustrations and fears. Perhaps you'll want to make regular appointments with your minister—at least at first—or another competent helping person. Don't keep your feelings bottled up because you feel ashamed of them. For you, too, a sense of family is vital. Different aspects can be provided in a variety of ways—through members of a support group or through your church.

Consistent fellowship with God provides the best sense of family. You may not have time for lengthy devotional times, but you can listen to tapes while you feed the baby and pray while you straighten the kitchen.

How do I deal with people who tell me that if I had enough faith, God would heal my disabled daughter?

Don't feel you need to convince these people that they are wrong. But you do need to know what you believe about the subject so they don't throw you off balance emotionally or spiritually.

Keep in mind that faith is not a disembodied quality or attitude that Christians should pump in themselves. Faith is firm trust in God as He is revealed in Scripture. Faith in "the King eternal, immortal, invisible, the only God" (from I Timothy 1:17) grows naturally as we know Him better.

From the Old Testament, the story of Job shows that it isn't faith that heals, but God who heals. And in some cases God allows a physical condition to remain in order to accomplish a higher purpose. Scripture taken in totality shows that not everyone will be physically healed in this life. A great deal, however, is said about suffering as a natural part of life in a world separated from God.

Human beings want to control their environment because they feel insecure when they can't. Finding someone to blame—many people don't dare blame God!—seems to solve their problem. Kindly but firmly state your position and don't let others heap guilt on your head.

How do I find a support group?

Talk with a social worker at the hospital, your physician, nurses, or others on the medical staff. Most hospitals have a list of organizations dealing with various disabilities and also names of parents of children with these disabilities who are willing to help others. Ask one of them to contact you and provide the information you seek.

Another option is to find local public organizations such as the library or department of health that have lists of such organizations. (See the Bibliography for national parent groups and agencies that will put you in touch with local support groups or individuals with whom you can network. Chapter 5 contains specific information about support groups.)

What is an advocate and should I have one for my child?

An advocate is a person who stands up for the rights of another. An advocate for a handicapped child is someone who would become informed about the rights and the services to which he or she is entitled. (For more information see the Bibliography in this book.) Resources are available through public and private agencies that may provide better quality life for your child. Part of an advocate's job is to locate the appropriate resource and persist in working with the proper individuals until the child's needs are communicated and proper action is taken. Usually one of the parents serves as the advocate for a handicapped child.

Being an advocate is harder for people who are naturally reticent and not used to taking initiative. (Caution: Assertiveness will accomplish more than aggressiveness.) But even if you are naturally shy, you, more than anyone else, realize how vital it is to act as a representative for your child in practical ways— getting medical information, locating the best therapist, etc. Suppose your child needs an important piece of equipment to help him or her develop physically, and you can't afford to buy it. To get it, you'll have to research and explore alternatives.

There are several parent coalitions that inform families of their rights and help them communicate effectively with the professionals involved in their children's lives. Other groups train parents to be advocates for their children. (Names of these groups are listed in the Bibliography.)

Our other children resent all the time it takes to care for Jeff who has muscular dystrophy. What can we do?

Have you explained Jeff's condition to them as simply as possible? Have you made sure they see him as a member of the family and not as a stranger who has taken Mom and Dad away from them? While it's detrimental to expect siblings to assume too much responsibility for Jeff, they do need to contribute to his care and feel part of his life.

Since Jeff will inevitably take a large part of your time, it's important that he not always be the center of attention. It is tough to maintain a balance. Some of these ideas may help:

- *Hold family meetings for family fun and communication.* Pick a time, such as after supper, when family members are generally in a good mood. Include a time when everyone can air grievances without censure. Employ problem-solving skills to come up with solutions to problems that affect the family.
- *Parent by appointment.* Plan for Dad to take one of the other children out for a hamburger one evening. Mom can do the same with another child while Dad baby-sits. Plan to do this on a regular basis.
- *Have realistic expectations.* As Jeff matures and develops, expect him to contribute to daily life however he can. Don't be shocked or overreact if his siblings resent him from time to time and don't want to be with him.
- *Use money fairly.* If all extra money goes for Jeff's special needs, family members will resent it. Start a fund, no matter how small, for your other children's recreation.
- *Learn to read your other children's behavior.* Long periods of silence, acting out inappropriately, or an overly responsible attitude, may be their ways of saying, "I need help in dealing with this." They may need to talk out their feelings with an understanding counselor.

People stare and make thoughtless remarks when I take my son who has cerebral palsy out in public. How do I deal with that?

All parents want their children to be accepted, handicapped or not. Public stares usually grow out of inexperience with disabled people. Inexperience results in curiosity and sometimes fear. Inexperienced people stare at *any* handicapped person. As more disabled people are mainstreamed into society, that attitude is changing.

If you are naturally shy, this may be a bigger problem for you. Be prepared with a simple, brief explanation of your son's condition to give to honest inquiries—especially those by children. Most of all, your own acceptance of your child, your obvious love for him, will set others at ease.

To some degree, stares and remarks are something that anyone who is different will always have to contend with. You can set the tone now so that your son can deal with these things in a relaxed, matter-of-fact manner later on.

My husband and I used to be close, but since the birth of our daughter Michelle, who is brain damaged, we've grown apart. What can we do?

Start to talk to each other about your feelings. Listen, really listen to what your spouse is saying, and pray for understanding. Remember, you are basically the same people you were before this crisis. The person who held feelings in will continue to do so now; the one who was demonstrative will act that way in this situation. The way each of you is acting is natural for you.

But a crisis exposes things about ourselves—"chinks in our armor"—areas of weakness that need special work. You may need marriage counseling to shore up places in your relationship that were shaky before but may have become worse because of the present stress. Such counseling can help you cultivate better communication skills which will be vital for maintaining your relationship.

Your need for personal growth is greater now than ever, so don't allow yourselves to become spiritually bankrupt. You can only encourage your partner if you yourself remain rooted in Jesus Christ.

Time alone together is essential. Look to family, friends, church members, or a local respite care agency to make this possible. Begin to see each other as people again—as man and wife—and not merely parents of a handicapped child.

If communication seems hard, maybe it's because one or both of you hasn't worked through the grief process. Guilt or anger, for example, may be so strong that it's interfering with your relationship. This is one time when it's crucial for you both to talk things over with a counselor.

My husband says I indulge our daughter and that she needs to be disciplined. How do you discipline a handicapped child?

While it may seem like a natural thing to do, indulging a handicapped child is not in their best interest. It may appear "cruel" to do otherwise, but remember that discipline is not punishment. Although at times it includes punishment, *discipline* means to train in order to develop self-control and character. That's your goal. You also want to help your child develop the skills necessary to remain safe and to function successfully in society.

Emotions and feelings of guilt often interfere. "How can I say 'no' to my blind or deaf child?" I might ask. I can do it because I love her and want her to become as well adjusted as possible. An indulged child may grow up expecting society to cater to her the way Mom and Dad did.

You may need to learn special techniques. A mentally retarded child, for example, will need rules repeated over and over.

When it comes to discipline, God can be our pattern. "God disciplines us for our good" (from Hebrews 12:10). Inevitably, my child will object the same way I object when God disciplines me. "No discipline seems pleasant at the time, but painful. Later on, however, it produces a harvest of righteousness and peace for those who have been trained by it" (Hebrews 12:11).

Pray for wisdom. Enroll in parenting classes for families with special children. Read literature about raising your child; talk with your pastor and other helpers; find out how parents in your support group have handled situations like yours.

We simply can't pay for all the doctor bills, special equipment and medication our handicapped son needs. What can we do?

There are a variety of resources available. Private agencies such as Easter Seals and the Muscular Dystrophy Association provide adaptive equipment for disabled children. Agencies like these have other services available for particular disabilities.

You will also want to investigate government agencies that provide aid. The Crippled Children's Services is a joint federal/state program to provide medical and related services to handicapped children from birth to age 21. Medical diagnosis and evaluation is provided free of charge; the range and cost of additional treatment or hospital services vary from state to state.

Look into aid that may be available from Supplemental Security Income, Medicaid, Social Security Disability Insurance Benefits, and Vocational Rehabilitation (federal and private), an organization that helps handicapped people become employable. (More information on these programs can be found in chapter 7.) There may also be resources funded on the state and local level. Check your local health department for guidance, too. Services vary from state to state and from case to case.

Another possible source of help is Shriner's Hospitals, located in several locations around the country. There, at no charge, a wide variety of in- and outpatient help is provided for those who qualify for their care.

God cares about these financial needs just as He cares about our other needs. Form the habit of committing them to Him. (Read Matthew 6:25-34.) Expect Him to guide you.

My husband and I keep asking ourselves what will become of our handicapped daughter if something happens to us?

Investigate options available as your child matures and make plans for her care. The option you choose will depend on factors determined by a complete evaluation of her total needs.

Options include supervised apartment living for those completely or partially self-supporting, residential care homes, and group homes. Ruth McEwen, counselor to handicapped people and their families (referred to in the Introduction of this book), believes some youth should be prepared for living in group situations when they become adults.

You'll also want to see if you're eligible for government aid. Families with financial resources sometimes opt to leave the bulk of their estate for the care of the handicapped offspring, explaining in advance to other members why they are doing so.

Doctors say my son will have a relatively short life because of his disability. How in the world can I live with this fact?

The Biblical view of life and death is far different from our earthly one. God Himself gives to all life and breath (Acts 17:25). When we die, we do not cease to exist but merely are changed from one state to another. Deformities, along with pain and suffering, are left behind. God is the One who decides what our life span on earth will be. Each of our days is a gift from God to us so that we may know Him and grow more like Him.

Certainly, you will experience emotional trauma. Family members can support one another by allowing each person to have down times. It complicates matters to expect unrealistic behavior and emotions from others.

As a family, live each day the way God intends for us to—live fully, experiencing together as much of the wonders of His world as possible. In doing so, you'll provide your son with a rich life.

In addition to your biological family, be part of your church family. Join a Christian care group for spiritual support.

Hope is essential. There is always the possibility that new treatment for his disability will be discovered. But most of all, hope in God, for He has promised that life is eternal. Remember, the disease doesn't control your child's life—God does. And He understands how you feel because He willingly allowed His own Son to live with the knowledge that He'd face an early, painful death.

CHAPTER FOUR

COUNSELING GUIDELINES

BARBARA WARD FED HER NEWBORN SON. HER OBSTETRICIAN *had just told her that he appeared to have Down's syndrome. "I convinced myself that I was holding a stranger, somebody else's infant," Barbara recalls.*[1]

When Paul Jablow's daughter Cara was born with the same condition as the Ward baby, he kept repeating to himself, "I have this feeling that Cara is dead. It's as if they took Cara away, the Cara who was just born to us, and replaced her with another baby." On the other hand, his wife Martha described herself as angry. When she held Cara, she'd look down in agony at the baby and scream silently over the unfairness of it all.[2]

Patty Kasnowski's son Ralph was born with a cleft palate. Where his mouth should have been, there was a gaping hole; part of his nose was also missing. Patty's first reaction was that her son didn't have a face at all.

Although she can't remember doing so, Patty cried out that she wished her son were dead. Now she firmly states, "Today, Brian is my life. But at the time, I rejected him. He just didn't look human."[3]

As these true accounts show, parents have a variety of intense emotional responses when confronted with the fact that their child is handicapped. The counselor or helper needs to be open to all kinds of responses and realize that they are normal.

The Counselors Own Feelings

Before the family can be helped, the counselor must examine his or her own attitudes toward the disabled. "Let's be honest," writes Donald Peake, whose two disabled children died shortly after birth and who is chaplain to people with developmental handicaps. "For the most part we see them as different—some less, some more, depending on the type and degree of their disability. . . . Moreover, we relate to these people largely in terms of their handicaps."[4]

Our own reactions may be even more extreme. If we've had little contact with people who have handicaps, we may feel afraid of them or even repulsed by their abnormalities. In the past, we may have avoided them and, consequently, doubt our ability to help. It's vital that we realize these feelings are normal—given our background and experience—and not sin or a weakness that automatically disqualifies us from helping.

Our feelings will likely change to ones of acceptance when we become informed about handicaps and gain experience with people who have them. Since these families are often among the most needy in the congregation, it is imperative that we pray for a healthy attitude and take steps to become comfortable with disabled people. We could visit local sheltered workshops, care facilities, and perhaps volunteer to help with Special Olympics or a similar activity in our area.

With education and experience we'll begin to realize the truth in what counselor Gary Collins points out: "It is rare to find completely handicapped people. While there are things which the handicapped person *cannot* do, there are also many things that he or she *can* do."[5]

A second important factor the helping person must assimilate is that the handicapped individual's personhood is intact despite the disability. He or she still reflects God's spiritual image, has a unique personality, characteristics, strengths, weaknesses, and abilities. (See Chapter 6 for more on the subject.)

Goals for Counseling Families of Handicapped

In order to counsel the family with a handicapped child, inform yourself about the particular disability. As physician Charlotte E. Thompson points out, the helper must also be able to empathize with the crushing pain the family feels. Great amounts of gentleness and patience are required because this pain doesn't go away easily. Some severely debilitating handicaps can grow progressively worse and, in some cases, be terminal. These situations are physically, emotionally, mentally, and spiritually depleting.

Here are some counseling goals, provided by people who are experts in the education and counseling of exceptional children:

- Help parents understand that the special child is a child first and a child with a disability second.
- Understand issues and facts related to the disability in order to help the child in the most constructive manner.
- Assist parents and the child to understand their feelings resulting from the disability.
- Aid parents and the child to accept the disability emotionally and intellectually without devaluing the individual possessing it.
- Help the child and parents to continue to develop their unique potentials together as a family and independently."[6]

Usually family counseling is necessary. Adjusting to the idea that a handicapped child has joined the family unit is necessary for father, mother, and each child. During counseling, help each person express their true feelings and thoughts. Guide them toward working together as a team.

Experts point out that two kinds of counseling are necessary. With the first kind, the helper provides the family members with the kind of information that will help them deal constructively with the situation. In the second, which is more difficult, the individuals explore their own feelings and attitudes and discover ways of resolving them.

Because of the severity of the initial crisis, it's impossible to determine how many sessions you'll have with the family. The degree of handicap of the child is a factor, as is preconditioning of parents.

Some come to the situation having weathered other crises, with strong inner reserves on which they can draw. Others, while not having had such experiences, are stable, mature Christians with unswerving faith in God. Still others, however, will be unstable in how they deal with these circumstances. For these the situation will be extremely difficult. Most people will be somewhere in the middle—average people with their own strengths and weaknesses.

First Objective: Console, Comfort, Encourage

You may become aware of the new crisis situation in a variety of ways—while visiting a new mother in the hospital, from a phone call notifying you of a child's accident, during a disabling illness, or following the parent's visit to a physician when they were informed that their child has a disability. Or perhaps the family is new to the church—they have lived with this for a while, but it's new to you.

Your goal on the first visit will be to console, comfort, and encourage. Parents use words such as *devastated, numbed, in shock* to describe their feelings when they first heard that their child was handicapped. "I fell apart," they may say. Or "I just couldn't believe it. I was sure the doctor had made a mistake."

They also may try to keep their composure for your sake. "I ask them where they're at, so they'll have an opportunity to tell me what they're *really* thinking and feeling," says Ruth McEwen, a counselor who specializes in those who are handicapped.

It's important to find out how the parents received the news. Was the physician sensitive when he told them? Were husband and wife together so they could support each other, or were they told separately? Was the news broken gently or dropped like a leaden ball on the floor?

In all likelihood, the parents will need more information about their child's handicap. Encourage them to learn as much as they can. They should ask their physician to explain the condition in layman's terms so they can understand. They could obtain lists from most hospitals of individuals who have a particular disability or parents of someone who has that condition. A visit from one of these people can be educational and reassuring. The caller may be able to put the parents in touch with a support group; if not, you provide the name and phone number of such a group. (See further information in Chapter 5.)

Let the parents tell you how they feel and listen carefully and sensitively. "My pastor helped me so much just by listening," parents say repeatedly.

One father told physician Charlotte E. Thompson that when he first heard his child was handicapped, he wished the child were dead—a response that badly frightened him. Try to see both parents together (unless the couple is separated). Provide reassurance that God has not abandoned them.

Ruth McEwen advises not only praying with the family but helping them so they can communicate with God on their own. It's important that, from the beginning, they depend on Him instead of letting their pain shut Him out. They may want you to read brief passages of Scripture reassuring them of God's presence and love that can remain with them when you are gone.

If the child is a newborn, ask if it's possible to see the baby. Some parents who haven't seen their child yet may suppose he or she is grotesque. You can help dispel that impression by commenting on positive qualities.

If these new parents haven't held their baby yet, and if it's medically feasible to do so except for their reluctance, your acceptance and encouragement may provide the impetus for them to take this important step. The sooner they hold the baby, the sooner the bonding process will begin, and acceptance will be expedited.

"It's important that they realize, as early as possible, that theirs isn't some different kind of creature, but a very real child with needs," McEwen says.

One of those needs could be immediate emergency surgery on the child. That means the parents will be asked to make quick decisions. If they're emotionally upset, that will be hard. You can help, not by making those decisions for them, but by acting as a sounding board. Encourage them to ask for as much time as possible to get their thoughts together and to be sure they understand the medical options, the purpose of the proposed surgery, the risks, and the potential gain.

A decision may have to be made about home versus institutional or other care. This decision rarely needs to be made immediately. Again, encourage the parents to obtain and consider all the facts first. Each situation must be weighed individually. Be sure to pray with them about this decision. An emotionally overwrought parent may opt for foster care or an institution (although fewer institutions are available today) and later decide to take the child home.

Find out on the initial visit what people from the church can do to help. Care for other children? Fix meals? Run errands? Help with housekeeping? Ask also if they would like visitors.

If the family is a member of the congregation, find out if you may tell other members about the baby's disability. People in the church will find it easier to provide the loving Christian support if they are given a little information. Be careful not to talk about the situation—not even to put it on the prayer chain if your church has one—until you have the parents' permission.

Promise to stay alongside the family as a helper. Reassure them of your love as well as God's, and remind them that they are not alone.

Remember to do some research about the disability as soon as possible. Be sure to investigate only current reliable sources since dramatic medical advances happen frequently. (Often information more than five years old is outdated and inaccurate.)

Because of the association of the family with your church, make opportunities or appointments to see them again. Offer to get together with them on a regular basis because some people are reluctant to ask for help even though they know they need it. Some couples feel that talking about the situation is just too painful. Yet they might agree to counseling if it was offered by someone in whom they have confidence and feel comfortable.

SECOND OBJECTIVE: HELP THE PARENTS TO GRIEVE.

Although they may not realize it, parents of a handicapped child often mourn the child they'd been expecting—the healthy baby who would fulfill their dreams.

Beatrice Wright points out the importance of this grieving process in the following statement: "One of the most pervasive conditions producing mourning is the inability or unwillingness of the person to sever ties with the endeared state that was. By mourning his loss, he brings the past into the present and in this way does not give up the past."[7]

Grieving is God's way of promoting healing, so individuals must be allowed and enabled to feel and express their responses as they occur.

The stages of grief through which many parents in this situation go are similar to ones described by Elizabeth Kubler-Ross in her book *On Death and Dying*. Not every individual experiences every stage. Some may pass through one stage quickly and linger in other stages.

In addition to the initial shock in these situations, people frequently experience the following five stages:

1. *Disbelief, denial, isolation.*

"It can't be true; there must be some mistake," they think—and withdraw from facts that are too painful. One mother described her denial stage like this: "Accepting the fact that my daughter is deaf has been very hard, especially since she had normal hearing until she had meningitis. In the beginning, I wouldn't even use the word *deaf*. Instead, I referred to her as *hearing impaired*. But Adrienne's audiograms show a profound hearing loss."[8]

Betty, the mother of two boys with cerebral palsy, pushed

doctors to evaluate her older son's condition because she knew something was wrong. "Finally when they say, 'You're right,' and give a diagnosis, you slip back into denial. Even though I was the one who initiated it, what I wanted was for them to look into [his condition] and say, 'Nothing's wrong.' "

Show parents examples from Scripture—that Job mourned his former state of health, wealth, and family; that Jeremiah grieved, and so did David—in order to give them *permission* to grieve as well, to let them know it's okay to feel this way.

They may have to experience grief numerous times. "Every month, you find out something new," Betty said.

The father of a multihandicapped child added, "It's as though you stand up and, *wham*, they knock you down. You may get up faster each time, but you drop further."

Some people act out the denial stage by refusing to accept an informed diagnosis, even after receiving several expert opinions that agree. Others simply refuse to acknowledge their disabled child, or, if they do provide care, they deny him or her the love that's needed.

Matthew Linn and his brother Dennis, write in *Healing Life's Hurts* that denial "is a necessary response to bring back emotional health and should not be fought."[9] Denial enables us to postpone dealing with hurts until we're ready. Too much, though, can prevent us from becoming whole again.

As parents receive accurate information about their child's condition, help them learn to focus on the child as a person and not merely on the disability. As they have physical contact with the child and establish a relationship, they will make the greatest strides through this stage.

2. *Feelings of Anger.*
During this stage, it's not uncommon for parents to rage at themselves, their mate, a physician, or any person who might have prevented a disabling accident or illness. Here's what one father wrote after he discovered his son was born blind:

"God, You seem very far from me right now. . . . Today I'm very angry, the angriest I've ever been at You. You know how much I have wanted a baby. I've prayed the baby would be born healthy. Well, God, he's blind. . . . It isn't fair, God. I do blame You for this loss."[10]

Angry parents ask questions. Questions like these: How could this happen to me? How can a loving God permit a child to be born in this condition. Here, the helper can discuss with them Scriptural answers to their questions about the meaning of suffering. (This issue will be thoroughly covered in Chapter 6.)

The angry person needs to see that anger isn't wrong—it's a response to a real or perceived injustice. But unchecked, it can lead to wrong actions—the angry person may lash out and cause deep, sometimes permanent wounds in family relationships.

Since anger is a difficult emotion with which to deal, counselors use different techniques. Some, such as the Linn brothers, have found inner healing methods successful in their work. Dr. Richard P. Walters, counselor and former staff psychologist in the adult outpatient department of Pine Rest Christian Hospital in Grand Rapids, Michigan, suggests several steps. Among them are these:

- Individuals must become aware of their anger.
- To the extent that it's possible, the individual must try to undo any damage the anger may have caused.
- After evaluating the situation that provoked the anger, determine whether the appropriate response should be resolution or indignation.
- Help individuals take steps to keep anger from growing. You might want to use this suggestion: "Ask yourself whether you are looking for a fire extinguisher or fanning the flame. Look for attitudes or internal messages that keep it going."[11]
- Individuals need to tell God and other appropriate people that they choose to deal with their anger constructively.
- Take the initiative to make the situation better.
- Forgive others *and* yourself. Without a doubt, Walters says, this is the most important part of the resolution of anger.[12]

Anger motivated Christ to cleanse the temple; and anger can spur parents to search out ways to help their disabled children. Karlee (Her story is told in Chapter 2.) says she became angry when she realized there were group homes for other people who needed them but not for those with head injuries. She knew from talking with parents like herself who had a head-injured older child that there was a need. If parents could no longer provide their care, the only alternative was a nursing home among elderly residents. It was Karlee's anger that energized her to spearhead plans that culminated four years later in the dedication of a residence in her city for the head-injured.

3. *Bargaining—attempting to make an agreement.*
Usually this means bargaining with God. "I'll accept my child as deaf—*if* she learns to read lips and speaks so she appears normal." "I'll accept my retarded son—*if* he achieves a higher level of ability than people predict."

The two Linns compare moving out of the bargaining stage to the young child who leaves crawling for walking. "Many falls, tears and a bruised nose testify that two feet don't offer the stability of creeping . . . . Eventually the day arrives when we can't angrily blame hard floors for our aches and pains but start blaming our own wobbly legs."[13]

The three steps they suggest in dealing with bargaining can be applied also to *each* phase of the grieving process: (a) the individual tells Christ how he or she feels; (b) the person finds in Scripture times when Christ faced a situation that could have aroused the same kinds of reactions; (c) finally, the person learns to live out Christ's reaction.

4. *Depression.*
Nearly a year and a half after Heidi's seizure disorder began, her mother confessed that both she and her husband had slipped into depression. "It finally hit us that she may be this way all her life." They were in debt; and they were exhausted from caring for their child around the clock in addition to their other responsibilities.

The Linns define *depression* as "swallowed anger that will disappear if I can answer the question, 'Who or what is irritating me?' and then deal with my anger."[14]

Depressed people may act passively, Gary Collins points out. They may need to be gently urged to take action and then be encouraged when they do so.

The primary care giver, the person who has the most responsibility for caring for the disabled person, may need a good physical checkup. If the family hasn't contacted a support group yet, urge them to do so.

Perhaps the parents are so swamped with things to do that they feel overwhelmed. Here, the church can help by providing teams to baby sit, do housework, shop, etc. If parents have been so busy caring for the child, making a living, traveling to the facility where he or she is housed, and keeping the family together, they may not have found time for prayer and Bible study. As the helper, you can do so with them on a regular basis.

Parenting the exceptional child can crush the self-esteem of some. At first, they may see only the disability and lose sight of the fact that the child was created in the image of God and that his or her soul is intact and important to Him. (For more on the subject, see Chapter 6.)

Feelings of guilt can also contribute to depression. To blame oneself is natural, especially for people who think that God punishes sin and rewards obedience in this life and that poor health and disability are punishment.

Counselor Gary Collins points out that guilt may be appropriate or it may be inappropriate. In this case, guilt is appropriate if the parent's sin caused the disability; guilt is inappropriate if this is not the case. An example of appropriate guilt would be guilt that results when a child is born disabled because of the mother's substance abuse during pregnancy.

Collins urges counselors to keep the following concepts in mind when helping those who feel guilt:

A. *Understanding and Acceptance*—Guilt feelings hurt, he points out. The counselor shouldn't minimize or criticize the individual who has them.

B. *Insight*—People often can be helped if they have some understanding of the forces which are influencing them from within. Collins suggests asking questions—ones that will help them see the source of the feelings. Help them determine whether these feelings result from training or experience and whether or not the concepts behind them are Biblical.

C. *Education*—Re-education about unjustified guilt can take time. But counselees need to be able to distinguish between appropriate and inappropriate accusations.

D. *Repentance and forgiveness*—Even if the guilt is genuine, it may take time before the individual is ready to repent. Instead of coercing them to confess, the helper may have to work with them until they can understand and accept the principles of God's forgiveness.[15]

5. *Acceptance.*

This last stage of the grieving process means to receive the circumstances willingly, not merely resignation to the inevitable. It's unrealistic to think that most people will embrace their difficult situation wholeheartedly daily. But, as Dr. Thompson points out, acceptance comes slowly, only after parents have grieved and explored their fears and anxieties.

Referring to accepting her own condition as a paraplegic, Ruth McEwen says "I wasn't free until I could thank God that I'm this way." She tells other handicapped people to take that step by faith, even though they don't feel like it. If they do, she says, God will honor their act and bring them inner wholeness.

McEwen admits that doing so was one of the hardest things she's ever had to do. Not that, by thanking God for the condition, the individual is saying that God deliberately engineers disabled bodies, but that God can use even that which He did not directly cause for His own good. For this, each one of us can be grateful.

This principle applies especially to families of the handicapped. Family members need to verbalize this decision to accept the circumstances in a variety of ways—in prayer, by journal writing (a helpful exercise which can be used throughout the restoration process), by sharing it with another family member and/or spouse.

Acceptance isn't necessarily a once-and-for-all event. It is an attitude that grows day by day. Parents demonstrate acceptance by nurturing their children in heartfelt love and by reaching out to others in similar situations.

THIRD OBJECTIVE: MEETING SPECIAL NEEDS OF FAMILY MEMBERS

Needs of the husband and wife.

Fathers often find difficulty accepting the fact they have a disabled child. They may have dreamed that this offspring would carry on the family name and now must face the fact that this may not happen. "I have known of fathers who took one look at their kid and that's the last anyone sees of them," says Frances Cooke Macgregor, a consultant to a special disability unit at New York University Medical Center. Macgregor adds that it is not unusual for marriages to break up after the birth of a handicapped child.

While the father may feel personal responsibility that the child is handicapped, the mother may feel this even more so. She *bore* the child. If the disability occurs later in the child's life as the result of an accident or illness, the mother was probably responsible for the child's care. She may wonder if there is something she could have done to have prevented the disability.

Thus, you the helper can understand how spouses in these families can experience unusual stress. Here are some questions

to consider as you are guiding them individually and as a couple:
- What kind of marital relationship did husband and wife have before the crisis?
- Do the present circumstances suggest they need marriage counseling?
- Does the mother feel overwhelmed because she has most of the responsibility for child care?
- Does the father feel left out?
- Does the couple communicate effectively with each another?
- Do they have good parenting skills?
- Is this their first child?

Problems can arise simply from differences the couple has in the way each spouse deals with stress. Lauralee and her husband had a rift after their child was diagnosed as multihandicapped. "My husband is my complete opposite and doesn't show his feelings," she says. "I cried for months after our son's diagnosis. My husband finally told me, 'Stop crying.' " Couples often need help in adjusting to these differences.

Needs of the siblings.

One friend who has a mentally retarded brother wanted to make sure counselors understand how hard the situation can be on siblings. "They can feel left out because this new baby takes so much time and attention." Counselor McEwen tells clients to make learning exercises and therapy with the handicapped child a family affair and celebrate each achievement together.

Couples experienced in parenting a disabled child emphasize the importance of being sure siblings understand the handicap to the best of their ability. Some parents wish they hadn't expected so much help from young siblings. They also wish they would have worked harder to give their nondisabled children more quality time.

Counselors can help parents discover ways of doing that. Just as with parents, siblings may need special help in exploring their own feelings and adjusting to the new circumstances.

Even grandparents have needs.

Grandparents may need time, help, and prayer to accept the exceptional child who also has not fulfilled their dreams. The father of two handicapped boys said, "In our case, one set of grandparents would say, 'They'll be fine.' So we went overboard trying to convince them of the truth. We'd exaggerate our children's conditions and then internalize our own words. Finally, we realized it wasn't our responsibility to make them accept the boys as they are. We had to accept them ourselves and get on with doing whatever we could to help them.''

As you involve yourself and members of your church in ministering to the needs of families with handicapped children, be alert to the fact that more than the nuclear family may have trouble dealing with the situation. Members of the extended family may also need a caring, listening "ear" to help them work through their feelings.

No family responds perfectly. When some members are not able to cooperate enthusiastically, the others need to be encouraged to be patient and go on together, depending upon God. The most healthy attitude to promote is to emphasize the *whole* family's well-being, not just that of the special child.

Early in the counseling process, parents or whoever is caring for the disabled child, should be encouraged to act as an advocate for him or her. That means insisting on an informed diagnosis, locating agencies that offer informational and financial resources, joining a support group, obtaining adaptive equipment, and monitoring the education. You can help them get started by providing the names of agencies in your area to contact. (Suggested resources are listed in Chapter 8.)

Fourth Objective: Socialization of the Handicapped Child

Jerry Adler worried about taking his handicapped child, Max, out in public, but his fears were somewhat abated when the first person he met stopped and remarked, ''Hey, he's real cute!'' even though the infant had a tracheal tube.[16]

Not all parents are as fortunate. ''I'd like to post a sign on my daughter's wheelchair telling what's wrong with her,'' one mother admitted. ''It doesn't bother my husband, but it does bother me,'' another said speaking of stares and questions.

Help the family realize that there will always be some people who stare and ask questions—even rude questions—because they are uninformed and inexperienced about the situation. A good way to handle these situations is to take charge of them. If the parent accepts the child, he or she will create an atmosphere of acceptance.

As much as the energy level of the care giver and the physical condition of the disabled child allow, encourage the family to expose the child to many different social situations—excursions to the zoo, trips to shopping malls, birthday parties, concerts, church activities, etc. The more the child is allowed to integrate into normal activities, the more quickly healthy socialization will take place.

Counseling the disabled child.
The child who develops a disability later on inevitably experiences a variety of emotions. The child may be fearful because the future may seem uncertain. If health problems have never been a factor, the adjustment to a more limited life-style may be especially hard.

Tim began having seizures when he was a young adolescent. "I think he was scared," his mother reflected. "He's 16 now and hard to deal with. He's afraid he'll have a seizure in front of his friends. His male image is affected. Doctors won't sign the papers so he can get his driver's license."

The thoughtless barbs of others, the feeling of being "different"—these things can be difficult at an age when self-worth is precarious anyway. Tim, and other older disabled children, may be concerned about the kind of work he'll be able to do; he may be mourning the fact that he no longer can pursue the career he had planned; he may wonder if he can have a relationship with a member of the opposite sex. Tim will grieve over the loss of his former self just as his parents are. He will need the same help as they.

Help the older child build self-worth based on Biblical principles. These principles are usually very different from those of contemporary society. Redirect the child to discover and cultivate new abilities, perhaps by encouraging participation in church programs. Evaluate family attitudes toward the disability to see how they may be affecting the child's.

Teens with disabilities often experience frustration regarding their sexual feelings. But some adults assume youths with disabilities don't have these feelings. To deal with that issue, helpers will need to inform themselves about disabled people and their sexuality or refer the adolescent to someone who has expertise in this area.

Helping the child with a degenerative disease.

"The families I know that have been most successful with this hard task make each day count," says Dr. Thompson.[17] Days count most when they are seen from the eternal perspective. Life is everlasting, for "the gift of God is eternal life in Christ Jesus our Lord" (from Romans 6:23). It isn't the number of mortal years that count, but our view of the nature and purpose of life. Here, the family can benefit by reflecting on Jesus' attitude during His time on earth.

Still, the emotional tension will be enormous. The helping person needs to be aware that depressive feelings will recur, especially as the child becomes weaker. These feelings will need to be talked out. A close relationship with God for all members of the family is vital. The knowledge of His presence and the solid promises of Scripture can provide unparalleled hope.

As their child grows, the family of the disabled child will face other crises. These include the child's transition into school (as early as two years of age in some states), entrance into adolescence; adjustment to a different system of receiving care, etc. At each stage, they'll have questions to ask and feelings to work through.

Counseling these families is extremely difficult. You, the helper, must not feel you have full responsibility for the successful adjustment of the family to this situation. The task is too big. You also don't want to be afraid to fail. If you should fail in some area, accept that fact, apologize, and try again.

You may come to a place where you feel you need to refer the couple and/or the child to someone who has more expertise in a certain area. It's always a good idea to not let yourself get in "over your head." Not every person is willing to receive guidance from another—maybe you feel someone else would be more effective in this situation. You want the best for everyone involved. Sometimes that requires flexibility and maybe even a little creativity.

There is a kind of failure, however, that should never happen, especially among Christians who are helping others—that is, promising to help but not following through. Be prepared for the temptation to withdraw when it nudges you, because working with these families requires an investment of time and emotional energy. As you try to answer the family's questions, you may be forced to deal with unanswered questions of your own.

Of all people in your church, families with disabled children are among the most vulnerable and in the most pain. Helping them can be some of the most rewarding experiences of your ministry.

Chapter Five

How the Church Can Help

DOES AIDING FAMILIES OF HANDICAPPED CHILDREN SOUND like a job you can't handle alone? It is! You'll need the assistance of a group—an extended family dedicated to accepting, nurturing, and discipling people of all kinds. In other words, you'll need the involvement of your whole church.

Helping handicapped children and their families is a task tailor-made for the Church of Jesus Christ. Different churches can help in different ways and to varying degrees, depending on their resources; you may want to consider joining forces with one or more nearby churches to implement some of the suggestions in this chapter.

Existing Support Groups

Your church can begin by referring families of disabled children to an established support group, if one exists in your area.

There are a wide variety of support organizations at the national, state, and local levels. Many of them provide information, training in raising disabled children, therapy, education, day-care centers, residences for community living, respite services, and recreational programs. Some put parents in touch with others whose children have similar disabilities, and help form local support groups. Not all services are available in all areas, however. For a list of organizations, see the Bibliography of this book.

Three of the most prominent national organizations offering help on a local level are Parentele, Pilot Parents, and the National Parent CHAIN (Coalition of Handicapped Americans Information Network). Each of these involves parents of children who have any type or severity of handicap.

Parentele is a national coalition created and operated by volunteer parents and friends. It links members, who include professionals and service organizations throughout the nation, in a communication system. This enables the group to give personalized information and promote parent-to-parent and professional contact. The *Crisscross* is its newsletter, in which members may place free classified advertisements.

Pilot Parents began in 1971 in Omaha, Nebraska. Its local groups train parents to help other parents of handicapped children in times of special need—when an initial diagnosis is made, for example.

National Parent CHAIN links existing parent coalitions, alliances, and other groups for information sharing purposes. It sends out timely information electronically and serves as a communication link between the state and federal governments. There are also a variety of national organizations designed to help those with specific handicaps. The National Information Center for Handicapped Children and Youth (NICHCY), which provided some information for this chapter, distributes fact sheets on specific handicaps. These sheets list names and addresses of national organizations as well as state chapters. The organization's state offices can provide information about chapters in your area. See the Bibliography for instructions on where to call or write for these fact sheets.

Families can also receive vital information and contact other parents in similar situations by using an information referral base. Stored in a computer, this information is updated regularly and includes such subjects as counseling available, residential treatment centers, aid programs, transportation, finances, and food stamps. Data can be called up on computer terminals which are part of the system. In my state, for example, a family could contact the University Health Science Center, which is linked with the system, to have questions answered—or to be put in touch with another family in a similar situation.

It's the local support group, however, that parents tend to depend on most. "When our son was born, the doctor put us in touch with the [support] group's president," a father told me. "She's been through it with her son. We talked things through and asked questions like, 'Who do we see for help?' and she had answers." He and his wife joined the group.

Joan Simon, mother of an autistic daughter, comments: "Much of what I have learned I've learned from other parents . . . I would say that involvement in a parents' group has been vital to our welfare."[1]

If such a group exists in your area, you should be able to find it through a physician or therapist, a local hospital, school district, sheltered workshop, social services agency, or a national organization listed in the Bibliography.

A Group of Your Own

If you're unable to find an established support group in your area, or if families of disabled children in your church would like a group that includes a distinctly Christian emphasis, what can you do? Your church may be able to sponsor a support group of its own, or in cooperation with other area fellowships. This could mean helping to bring parents together, providing a meeting place, donating or loaning supplies and equipment, finding a leader, or formulating guidelines to get started.

In my city, one church provides a meeting place for a support group. The group was started by three mothers who have disabled children. Each mom had found a different therapy program—and was unaware that the other programs existed. Wanting to spare other parents the struggle they'd gone through to find help, the women pooled their information and put together a list of resources. Out of that beginning came an organization which, thanks to donations, provides therapy for those who couldn't otherwise afford it. The organization sponsors the support group, which meets monthly.

If your church decides to sponsor a group, here are guidelines that may be helpful. Some are based on those suggested by Bette M. Ross in the book *Our Special Child* (Walker, 1981).

Getting members. If you have one or two families in your church who are interested in forming a support group, you might find others by placing a newspaper ad describing your project. Include a telephone number inquirers can call. The person who answers the phone should be ready with a date, time, and place for the first meeting.

Medical personnel and social service agencies probably won't give you names and addresses of parents who might be interested, but might be willing to contact the parents themselves. Or you may be given permission to post information on a bulletin board or include it in a mailing. Other churches in the area may be willing to let parents of disabled children in their congregations know about the meeting. The founders of your group will, of course, have to decide ahead of time whether all disabilities or just one will be represented in the group.

The first meeting. Help everyone feel as comfortable as possible. Some groups serve tea and coffee during an initial social time to create a relaxed atmosphere. Ask parents to introduce themselves to the group and to tell a little about their children if they wish.

Next, ask questions that will prompt group discussion. For example:
- How did you first learn your child had a disability?
- Was the information you received at that time adequate?
- What kind of treatment is your child receiving, and are you satisfied with it?

Maintain an atmosphere in which parents will feel accepted no matter what they say. Group goals should be set, too. Ask what individual parents' goals for their children are; out of these a group goal may eventually emerge.

Before the meeting is over, get a list of participants' names and addresses. Set a regular meeting date. Encourage those present to invite others who'd like to attend.

Future meetings. Bette Ross suggests going slowly so that participants get to know each other. While major goals are taking shape, set small ones such as raising money for initial supplies. Decide where meetings will take place. Make arrangements for baby-sitting.

Eventually, leaders will emerge from the group and an organizational structure will be established. If the group wants to be tax exempt, the leaders can follow steps listed in *Our Special Child.*

"Remember that a parent group is a caring group," writes Bette Ross. "Taking care of each other, being genuinely concerned about each other, sharing the good and bad will strengthen the family feeling of your club."[2] One way to maintain contact, she suggests, is to appoint a telephone chairperson who calls absent members to see whether a child is ill or whether there is another emergency.

Members of the group can help each other deal with the depressions and frustrations of parenting the disabled. They can share the knowledge gained through the experience of handling practical matters. The group can also invite local professionals to address the membership on such subjects as how to obtain financial help and how to act as advocates for disabled people.

Church leaders can also be invited to address the importance of a strong spiritual base. Counselors can provide ways to cope with the mental and emotional anguish. Films are also available, but make sure the ones you show are up-to-date and well done.

To stay vital, the group will need to help parents of both disabled infants and older children. One mother dropped out of a support group because it concentrated only on the needs of new mothers; her child was reaching adolescence. "I could tell them how I coped with the early years," she said, "but no one could help me with my problems now." Keeping in mind the changing crises families face through the years, try to provide varied resources and guided discussion groups.

Possibilities for other group activities abound. Members may want to publish a newsletter, for example, or train volunteers who can be called on to visit new parents of disabled children. The group's purposes can be elaborate or simple, but one thing needs to remain clear: The group exists to comfort, inspire, inform, and provide hope and a sense of togetherness to parents and other caretakers—so that they and their disabled children can have the best possible quality of life.

Seeing that happen is the reward for those who work hard to get such a group going. I saw that pleasure on the face of one such person, a father whose two sons have cerebral palsy. He'd just returned from answering the phone.

"It was the mother of 11-month-old twins," he reported. "Just today, one of them was diagnosed as being mentally retarded. A nurse in the hospital told [the new mother] about this group. She was very relieved just to talk with me for a few minutes." He added, "Hopefully, she'll be a little better off than we were because she has someone to talk with who's been there."

The Church As Support Group

Is a support group of crisis-stricken families enough? No. A second, equally vital support system is that of the church.

Why? First, a family may or may not have a parent or parents who can cope with the situation. Spouses may not even be able to support one another. Single parents, too, must face the crisis alone. A spiritual family is needed, one that makes its presence known in visible, tangible ways.

Even if families could somehow survive on their own, Christians would still be exhorted by the New Testament to show their faith in acts of love toward needy members of the Body of Christ. "As we have opportunity, let us do good to all people, especially to those who belong to the family of believers," writes Paul to the Galatians (6:10). Jesus Christ Himself set down the principle. "The Son of Man did not come to be served, but to serve" (Matthew 20:28).

How can a local church support its families who have disabled children? To begin at the beginning, it can welcome the newborn disabled child in the same way it would others born to members of the congregation. Is it customary in your church to put a rose on the pulpit for a new baby or to send flowers to the hospital? If so, be sure to do that for parents of a child with a disability, too. List the child on the cradle roll if that's a custom in your church. Arrange to have someone in the nursery who can care for the child.

Members of the congregation may not know how to act toward the family. Some may keep their distance; others may make well-intended but inappropriate remarks. They need guidance. As the Reverend Robert V. Thompson once said from the pulpit of the First Baptist Church in Granville, Ohio, "Aren't we afraid of what we see mirrored in the handicapped? We don't know what to do with them. We can't cure them. They need to be taken care of. But worst of all, they reflect the finitude, the boundaries, the limits of life. We hate to face our own limitations. Yet, maybe we can learn something when we face our own limits."[3]

Church leaders can help congregations by providing literature about disabilities. Check the organizations listed in the Bibliography for the material you need. Try featuring books on the subject in your church library. Pamphlets describing ways to relate to disabled people could be placed in the foyer or another easily accessible area.

Some churches schedule a "Handicap Awareness Sunday," too. Such an event may be prompted by the fact that a disabled person has joined the congregation, but it shouldn't focus on that person; the disabled in general should be discussed. Experts from the community may be invited to speak, and the pastor could present a sermon on God's attitude toward those with disabilities and their place in the church. You could also follow the example of one pastor who invited several disabled adults, acting as a panel, to answer questions from the congregation.

Down-to-Earth Help

During the initial crisis—the disabled child's birth, the diagnosis, or a disabling accident—the family will need practical help. This includes bringing in meals, assisting with housework, providing child care (for the disabled child and/or other siblings), helping with the shopping, providing transportation, and giving financial help. A child may also need an advocate from the congregation if the parent(s) can't perform this role.

How can your church be sure these needs are being met? One way is to appoint a coordinator—a person to whom care givers go when a need arises. The coordinator can keep a list of volunteers—people willing to do specific jobs for the family. The coordinator might be an adult Sunday School class representative, a member of a women's group, or a close friend of the disabled child's family.

Help with home therapy is one need that may arise soon after the birth or accident. In one community, friends and neighbors signed up to perform patterning— exercises designed to help brain-damaged people—with a disabled child.

Another couple, Roseanne and Jordan Peckin, wrote the nearly 100 people who volunteered to help "pattern" their son Matthew: "Our son thrives and prospers . . . because of you."[4] Volunteers manipulated his body and taught him colors, shapes, words, and numbers. In four years Matthew learned to crawl and creep, to read and feed himself.

Most therapy programs don't require as many people or hours. But volunteers from the church may be able to help with a more modest program, or do other chores so that parents are free to give time to therapy. Like the people who volunteer to help Matthew, they'll find that doing so changes their lives for the better.

A Place to Grow

The dedication or baptism of an infant is a thrilling occasion for most Christian parents. The family of a child with a disability should be invited to participate in whichever ceremony your church performs. There is no need to distinguish between this and other babies in the presentation. Emphasize the child's value to God and his or her place in the Christian family.

During most ceremonies of this type, the congregation is challenged to model Christlikeness as the child grows, to help lead him or her to a saving knowledge of Christ, and to assist parents in rearing him or her in the nurture and admonition of the Lord. But the congregation cannot meet that challenge unless it makes a special effort to do so.

Suppose, for example, the child is deaf. Does anyone in the church know sign language? Are there Christians in the congregation who are willing to learn it? They can do so by registering in a sign language program sponsored by a local community college or other agency. Church leaders may choose to interpret an existing Sunday School class and worship services, or to set up a separate class for the deaf.

What if your church has only one child who has a particular disability? As you consider whether to start a special program for that child, try to find out whether there are others in your community who have a similar disability but are unchurched. Could they join? Even if you can find only one child, doesn't he or she deserve the opportunity to receive an effective spiritual education? And if your church can't sponsor a special program, can other churches help?

Children with differing handicaps will need specialized help to learn. Flannelgraphs won't help a blind child, for example. Why not appoint a committee to research the best ways to teach children whose handicaps are represented in your congregation? Have the group report to the church's Christian Education committee. The committee may also want to look into ways to communicate the Gospel to children whose handicaps are not now represented, in order to be prepared for the future. Meanwhile, you can assign a tutor or helper to a disabled child who has recently entered the church.

The committee can also find out whether the child with a disability can be included in the church's regular camp. Are facilities accessible? Is there an interpreter for the deaf? The committee can also locate special camping programs for children with handicaps. Further, the group can link parents, Sunday School teachers, Bible club leaders, and youth directors, suggesting resources that may help.

Teachers and youth workers aren't the only ones who'll have to know how to communicate with the disabled child. The rest of the congregation will, too, if it's to relate to the child as a spiritual family. Members of the congregation can use gestures and notes to communicate with a deaf child, perhaps even learning a few words in sign language. They can be told how to help a mentally retarded child participate in a game at a church picnic, or to see that a child in a wheelchair is centrally located rather than always stuck on the fringes. Relating to a child with a disability can be catching; when a few people do it unself-consciously and openly, others are likely to follow suit.

An older disabled child will probably want to be included in the church's youth group activities. Leaders will probably need to confer with the adolescent's care givers and arrive at ways to accomplish this.

Able-bodied young people may need to be told how to relate to disabled youth, to feel comfortable with them so that they can make friends. When leaders do this, they should point out that most handicapped youth can do many of the things others can. The deaf can participate in sports, for example; those in wheelchairs can play games, though they may need help to adapt them.

One youth group member could be appointed to plan ahead so that disabled members can participate in group activities. For instance: When the young people go to a concert, are the facilities accessible to a wheelchair? If one of the group or a likely visitor is in a wheelchair, what arrangements can be made to accommodate him or her?

The same goes for your church's own facility. Are the disabled children in your church family—and those who may visit—able to enter and navigate the building? Are rest rooms adapted for the handicapped?

As you seek to sensitize your congregation to the needs and value of disabled people, you may want to use resources like Joni Eareckson Tada's two-part video series for children, *Let's Be Friends* and *Meet My Friends* (David C. Cook Publishing Co., 1988). The video and accompanying leader's guide are designed for elementary children, but could be used as part of a program to help able-bodied people of all ages understand and feel comfortable with the disabled.

You can help disabled children and their families feel that they are part of your church body by providing acceptance, a teaching program suitable for each child's needs, and opportunities for fellowship and participation. All this will take time, but most families will be pleased when they see your church making an honest effort.

Disabled Children Are Gifted, Too

As children grow, the church can help them discover, cultivate, and use their gifts and talents. One church, for example, assigns willing young people to work with mature adults as "apprentices." This may include disabled persons. Those interested in reading can assist the church librarian; those who like electronics can help the person who handles the sound system; those with musical inclinations work with someone on the music committee.

If members of the congregation think about the disabled child in terms of what he or she *can* do, they will naturally find ways to let him or her participate. A mentally retarded child could help set the table for a church potluck, collect bulletins left on pews after church, or sharpen pencils for the pew racks. A deaf child might take the offering; one in a wheelchair could read Scripture or lead a class in prayer.

Sunday School department heads can ask parents or children about interests and abilities, then find ways to let the children contribute. An artistic child might arrange the bulletin board; one who likes to write could contribute to the church newsletter. In some cases patience will be necessary, especially if the child is mentally handicapped and needs to be taught repeatedly how to do a job. Children should be allowed to make mistakes; after all, the goal is not to have an unflawed church program but to build people.

Helping Those Who Can't Attend

Parents and others who care daily for handicapped children need special consideration as well. Because their children may be sick often, they may not be able to attend church regularly. But a volunteer can see that they receive tapes of services they miss.

One church has a special service available to shut-ins via a telephone conference call. Those who "attend" this service feel they are participating even though they can't be there physically. Families of handicapped children might appreciate such a service if your church can make one available.

The disabled child who can't attend regularly may need to be taught Sunday School lessons at home by a teacher. Even if the child is institutionalized, he or she should not be dismissed as being no longer part of the assembly. Volunteers could help parents by visiting the child regularly if the institution is close enough, taking the child out for a drive if possible. The church could provide gifts for the child at birthdays and other holidays. Church leaders could find out whether the child receives spiritual instruction—and whether the church can assist in that.

A Long-Term Commitment

A congregation's commitment to a disabled child and his or her family is not a brief or easy one. If the child's health deteriorates, the family will need emotional support and prayer. The child and family, periodically frustrated over limitations or rejection or unfulfilled dreams, may withdraw or show signs of anger—and need understanding.

Generally, families of disabled children report that they do not find in churches the kind of support they need. "Most parents . . . may attend church for a few years, or until a religious milestone has been reached, but other than that, they don't expect much from the church for their disabled children—simply because most families haven't found it there," writes Bette Ross.[5]

That can change. The church can be the one place in which each child is accepted and loved. From the early crisis through therapy, from beginning school to adolescence, from vocational training to adulthood, we belong to one another. Our relationships with these families will do at least as much for us as for them. All that can happen when we live out this verse: "Be devoted to one another in brotherly love. Honor one another above yourselves . . . Share with God's people who are in need" (Romans 12:10-13).

Chapter Six

God's View of Handicapped People

"*HY DID A LOVING GOD INVENT A WORLD THAT INCLUDED spina bifida? Why doesn't He answer the prayers of all those who continually tell me they are praying?*"

Those are questions Steve Harris, pastor of Evangelical Baptist Church in Sharon, Massachusetts, asked himself when his son Matthew was born with that condition. Certainly, he has more reason than most for his Job-like "whys." Matthew has a severe degree of spina bifida, failure of the spinal column to properly form and close. A complication of that condition with which the Harris's have had to cope is apnea—periods when a person fails to breathe. "Our current estimate is that Matthew has stopped breathing and nearly died over 2,700 times."

In a conversation with a seminary friend, Harris agonized out loud about his dilemma: How could he recommend a loving God to others when he himself was barely on speaking terms with Him? He described himself as, on occasion, mouthing truths to his congregation about God's purpose in suffering that he simply didn't feel himself.[1]

Even the most theologically informed may have to start learning all over about suffering and God's purposes when "statistics" strike home—when a disability occurs to someone special to them. Now their questions about suffering aren't merely academic; they're personal, and they threaten the very core of their faith.

One way Harris found answers to his own questions was through a study of the Book of Job with an adult Bible class in his own church. He approached the study apprehensively because he knew he still hadn't dealt with all of his own anger. "Yet the teaching of that book, forcing myself to come honestly to God's perspective on suffering, was what first began to answer my questions and unravel my confusion."[2]

God's Viewpoint on Suffering

Apart from Scripture, there are no answers to questions families naturally ask—"How can a good God allow my child to go through life in this condition?" Not all of God's answers are like neat, computer printouts. Nor are they kindly assurances that God will "kiss it and make it well." The Bible doesn't specifically address the reason God allows children to have disabling handicaps. But it *does* say much about suffering.

It's important to distinguish between two kinds of "why?" questions. The first is: How can God allow children to be born with disabilities (or acquire them during childhood)? The second is: Why is God allowing this to happen to me?

Most parents search for personal answers to these questions in order to find peace in the midst of their circumstances. But for Christians, these answers must line up with God's truth as revealed in Scripture—not answers that merely "feel good" or can be found in the latest "pop" psychology book. Answers to life's dilemmas that are not founded on God's truth are like eating a dinner of doughnuts—you get full, but you're dissatisfied, even sickened, because what's been ingested is sugary, not substantial.

The Christian counselor can help by patiently guiding the individual to form a Biblical philosophy of suffering through personal study of God's Word and by asking questions—perhaps the same ones over and over—as he or she struggles toward acceptance of the situation much the same way Job did during his suffering. The helping person can use the Book of Job to assure the individual that asking "why suffering?" questions is not wrong; only charging God with wrongdoing and cursing Him is sin (Job 1:22; 2:9, 10). As these people explore their questions about suffering, they will learn principles that shed light on the second question as well—"Why is God allowing this to happen to me?"

Scripture cites several reasons why people suffer that apply to this situation. Here are a couple of them:

- *Sin has permeated our planet*. It began in Eden when Adam and Eve chose to disobey God (Genesis 3). The result of man's fall into sin is described by the apostle Paul: "We know that the whole creation has been groaning as in the pains of childbirth right up to the present time. Not only so, but we ourselves, who have the firstfruits of the Spirit, groan inwardly as we wait eagerly for our adoption as sons, the redemption of our bodies'' (Romans 8:22, 23).

The whole passage (verses 18-24) suggests that we live in a world in which malformation and decay is interwoven into the fabric of earth and its inhabitants because the world is separated from the source of perfection, God Almighty.

All people, Christian and non-Christian, are subject to the results of Adam's and Eve's fall into sin. As a consequence people experience death and deformity which are foreign to God's original plan. Although people are made new through rebirth, that regeneration takes place in a person's spirit. Physical bodies will be redeemed when salvation is completed—when believers in Jesus Christ as Savior, meet our Lord to be with Him forever.

Parents I spoke with vehemently oppose all suggestions that God causes disabilities—that He creates twisted bodies that result in decades of pain for the disabled person and the family. ''Not God,'' one father said emphatically, but ''nature'' caused this problem. In other words, he was not blaming God for his child's disability but the fallen condition of the world.

Another time the mother of a child with cerebral palsy put it this way. ''I'm part of a sinful world. That's why my child is this way. I've never said, 'Why me?' It's more realistic to ask, 'Why not me?' It's just the natural consequence of living in the world as it is.''

• *Suffering is permitted by God to reveal His glory.* At some point parents will wrestle with the idea that an almighty God could have prevented this from happening. *If He's so good and so powerful, then why didn't He?* The answer in Scripture is that God created an originally good environment. When Satan chose evil and influenced mankind to follow him, God set in motion His plan to provide mankind with a way back to fellowship with Himself through the death and resurrection of His Son, Jesus Christ. Now, even though evil is the ongoing state of the world, God is able to use that very evil for His long-term good purposes (Romans 8:28-30).

The ancients perceived suffering as punishment. In Jesus' day, ''suffering because of one's personal sin'' was the predominant theology about suffering, and the disciples reflected it. Once, when they met a blind man, one of Jesus' disciples asked Him,

''Rabbi, who sinned, this man or his parents, that he was born blind?'' (John 9:2). They reasoned that if a baby was born blind, it must be punishment for his parents' sin or else the baby had sinned in his mother's womb.

This reasoning was refuted by Jesus Himself. '' 'Neither this man nor his parents sinned,' said Jesus, 'but this happened so that the work of God might be displayed in his life' '' (verse 3).

This does not mean that a disability is never the result of someone's wrongdoing. A drunken parent driving a car that goes out of control and severely disables a child is an example. The injury in this case can be seen as the natural consequence of the direct action of the parents.

Despite Jesus' words, parents still heap guilt on themselves when none need exist. The father of a hydrocephalic (abnormal amount of fluid around the brain), cerebral palsied child, described his own struggle. ''My wife was pregnant when we came home from the mission field a year and a half before our term was up. When our child was discovered to be handicapped, I kept thinking maybe it was punishment because I hadn't stayed on the mission field for the whole term.''

It's not easy for parents or disabled adolescents to deal with guilt—real or false. Feelings of guilt can prevent God from using the situation constructively. It may take months or even years before they can fully rid themselves of the emotional wounds that guilt can bring. For some, healing seems to remain just out of reach. Counselors need to be cautious and sensitive where individuals are in the process.

It took Joni Earickson Tada years, after a diving accident at age 17 left her a quadruplegic, to see that this accident was permitted by God. But this disability has enabled her to minister in special ways to special people. Here's what Joni wrote after those years of questioning, praying, and searching:

''God deliberately chooses weak, suffering, and unlikely candidates to get His work done so that when the job is accomplished the glory goes to Him and not us. . . . He screens the suffering, filtering it through fingers of love, giving us only that which works for good and which He knows will point us to Him. As we grow in our faith, our way of looking at things changes. Once it seemed as if the only way God could glorify Himself would be to remove our sufferings. Now it becomes clear that He can glorify Himself through our sufferings.''[3]

C. S. Lewis's comments in *The Problem of Pain* further amplify the subject. "Suffering is not good in itself. What is good in any painful experience is, for the sufferer, his submission to the will of God, and, for the spectators, the compassion aroused and the acts of mercy to which it leads."[4]

Joni is an example of a person who went on to minister through her disability. Parents can, too, as they visit others who've just learned that their child is handicapped. Also consider people who've formed support groups that have become lifelines for many in their community—that, too, is an important ministry.

Even though they know that serious disabilities are part of life in this world, parents still have a right to pray for healing. "That God can and does, on occasions, modify the behavior of matter and produce what we call miracles, is part of the Christian faith; but the very conception of a common, and therefore, stable, world, demands that these occasions should be extremely rare," Lewis wrote.[6]

Counselor Ruth McEwen, disabled herself, reminds clients that, although Jesus healed many while He was here on earth, nowhere does the Bible state that He healed *all* (Mark 1:34; 3:10). Christian parents will pray for healing and may want their child to be prayed for by the pastor or elders of their church. But unless they're prepared to see that their hope rests in God alone and not in healing, the experience could lead to depression if healing doesn't occur. That's what happened to one parent who finally gave in to pressure and took her child to a visiting faith healer.

Parents such as these can be helped to identify with Paul, who prayed three times that his "thorn in the flesh" would be taken away. Each time God seemed to say "no." Here is how the Lord responded to Paul's request: " 'My grace is sufficient for you, for my power is made perfect in weakness.' Therefore I will boast all the more gladly about my weaknesses, so that Christ's power may rest on me. That is why, for Christ's sake, I delight in weaknesses, in insults, in hardships, in persecutions, in difficulties. For when I am weak, then I am strong" (II Corinthians 12:8-10).

Use Scriptures About Healing Carefully

Another way to help is to provide resources or guidance so

parents can understand and interpret Scriptures about healing. Sometimes well-meaning family members and friends may quote from passages that may have been taken out of context. Is a meaning being read into the verse that the text doesn't support? The Bible says that God moves mountains, but the passage doesn't imply that He chooses to move every mountain.

Check to see if the people you are helping may be reasoning from a Biblical premise but using faulty logic. Does their theology concerning *faith* seem sound? Do they regard it as a quality they must somehow "get" on their own? Or do they consider it to be an ability to trust God that begins as a choice but grows as they get to know Him better? Do they realize that God heals according to His sovereign will?

People Can Distort Individual Worth

In addition to a Biblical philosophy of suffering, families of disabled children need a Biblical view of human worth. An inaccurate perception of individual value may cause a handicapped child to be rejected and may seriously affect the child's sense of esteem.

One mother said, "My husband's family hasn't accepted our handicapped child. Such things don't happen in their family is what they seem to be saying. They even suggested that their son isn't the father of this child."

Our society places such a high premium on physical perfection that there is a tendency to view the exceptional child as flawed and therefore devalued. So it's no wonder that, in some cases, those involved have a hard time seeing disabled people as acceptable and worthwhile.

Often the person who has the most difficult time realizing value in a disabled child is someone who possesses a poor sense of self-value and identity. This means that even family members may have a difficult time valuing the disabled child—an older son because his brother or sister is "different" from his peers' siblings; the parents who birthed the child because she resulted from their union. These attitudes may also include extended family.

How can you help these people? First of all, pray for wisdom. Then gradually shift their gaze from the world's system of value and worth to God's. Help them rethink what "normal" means. (After all, their child has been branded as "abnormal.") Upon closer examination, they'll see that the word *normal* means "conforming to the accepted standard," and that's a highly ambiguous concept. Point out that everyone has some kind of flaw, although it may not be as noticeable or severe as those of the disabled child.

This kind of rethinking will take time. But the individual who comes to realize that it's God, not people, who gives a person worth can begin to see himself or herself, as well as others, through God's eyes and can experience divine love and acceptance through the embrace of the Christian community. A big step toward emotional and spiritual wholeness will have been climbed.

Occasionally you may encounter someone who tries to support a misperception of handicapped people by claiming that God regards disabled people as second-class citizens. This person may try to base this on the fact that in the Old Testament members of the tribe of Levi who were handicapped were not allowed to serve in the Temple.

These people are failing to understand the Biblical context of those circumstances. This period was under the Law, the Old Covenant, when righteousness was typified ceremonially through externals. Even animals brought for sacrifice had to be without blemish. This ceremonial requirement did not mean God devalued the individual Levite but that physical "spotlessness" was symbolic of the perfect Redeemer who was to come.

God's View of Value of Persons

Under the New Covenant, however, internal holiness, not ceremonial external perfection, is what is required. In addition to providing personal "spotlessness" through redemption, our Lord corrected the misconception that had developed in contemporary thought about a person's value based on physical characteristics. As the Incarnation of God, Jesus showed particular concern for handicapped people; He paid special attention to them, reflecting God's own attitude toward them.

Throughout the Old Testament, the Scriptures are filled with passages that reveal God's attitude toward the suffering of His people. For example, when the Israelites were helpless slaves in Egypt, God said, "I have indeed seen the misery of my people in Egypt. I have heard them crying out because of their slave drivers, and I am concerned about their suffering. So I have come down to rescue them . . . '' (Exodus 3:7, 8).

The prophet Jeremiah tells more about God's compassion. "Because of the Lord's great love we are not consumed, for his compassions never fail. They are new every morning; great is your faithfulness. I say to myself, 'The Lord is my portion; therefore I will wait for him' '' (Lamentations 3:22-24).

Compassion and loving-kindness toward all are attributes of God's nature. In addition He values people—Jew or Gentile, slave or free, male or female, *and* able or disabled. The apostle Paul expresses God's view of the worth of individuals by citing ways He demonstrates His love:

[He] has blessed us in the heavenly realms with every spiritual blessing in Christ. For he chose us in him before the creation of the world to be holy and blameless in his sight. In love he predestined us to be adopted as his sons through Jesus Christ, in accordance with his pleasure and will . . . . In him we have redemption through his blood, the forgiveness of sins, in accordance with the riches of God's grace that he lavished on us with all wisdom and understanding. . . . In him we were also chosen . . . in order that we . . . might be for the praise of his glory. . . . [We were] marked in him with a seal, the promised Holy Spirit, who is a deposit guaranteeing our inheritance until the redemption of those who are God's possession—to the praise of his glory (from Ephesians 1:3-14).

By absorbing these truths deep into his or her spirit, the parent who feels inferior because a child is less than perfect and the older disabled child who denigrates himself or herself for the same reason, can find inner healing. "The Lord does not look at the things man looks at. Man looks at the outward appearance, but the Lord looks at the heart" (I Samuel 16:7).

I am not worthwhile because of what I look like or what I can accomplish. *I am worthwhile because God values me.* It is the spirit of a person and godly character qualities that are the essence of true beauty.

We must help people remember that, although physical imperfections may seem objectionable to the standards of our culture today, they are merely temporal. Christ himself was disfigured with stigmata, a fact that can assure families even more that He understands their situation. "So we fix our eyes not on what is seen, but on what is unseen. For what is seen is temporary, but what is unseen is eternal" (II Corinthians 4:18).

If families are careful to base their views of disabled children on Biblical principles, they will realize that these special children deserve the same dignity and respect as all people. It's vital that they continue to see these children from God's perspective, because, by inference, some dispute the personhood of handicapped infants—especially those unborn. (The latter refers specifically to the fact that some justify abortion if it can be determined that the fetus has a defect. Amniocentesis, a technique to make this determination, was mentioned in Chapter 1.)

For instance, author Steven Baer, writing in *National Review,* takes issue with Judge Gerhard Gesell's statement that "some infants born with physical and mental defects may well fit within that broad definition of 'person' "—seeming to infer that not all do. "The fundamental tenet of law and medicine—of all society for that matter—is that which estimates the individual as of primary, sacred worth," Baer says.[6]

All Christians Are Gifted Members of the Body of Christ.

Here is another Scriptural principle families of handicapped need to grasp. As Paul wrote to the church in Corinth,

The eye cannot say to the hand, "I don't need you!" And the head cannot say to the feet, "I don't need you!" On the contrary, those parts of the body that seem to be weaker are indispensable, and the parts that we think are less honorable we treat with special honor. . . . But God has combined the members of the body and has given greater honor to the parts that lacked it, so that there should be no division in the body, but that its parts should have equal concern for each other. If one part suffers, every part suffers with it; if one part is honored, every part rejoices with it (I Corinthians 12:21-26).

Because the problem that apparently existed in Corinth can still be found today—giving preference to special, distinguished members—it is especially important for families to know for themselves what the Bible teaches about the status of so-called "weaker" parts. These parts contribute to the well-being of everyone within the Christian community.

Knowing this can help overcome some of the feelings parents have that at least some of their aspirations for their child will not be realized. A Down's syndrome daughter may not be an Ivy League graduate. But as a believer in Jesus, she's a member of His Body. That means she's gifted (Romans 12:6; I Corinthians 12:7), a fact some may struggle to accept.

I began to realize this truth when I started visiting a nursing home where some residents are mentally impaired. Always, they greeted me warmly—a broad smile and a hug. There are few places where a person can experience this kind of acceptance. I have come to believe that their unique, loving nature is a special gift from God from which the whole world can benefit.

The list of abilities with which God gifts His people is vast. One of the most astounding illustrations of special giftedness exhibited in a disabled person is found in Leslie Lemke. Severely retarded, blind, and crippled by cerebral palsy, Leslie began playing piano and singing at age 16 without any instruction. Now 34, he travels and gives concerts. "We believe what Leslie has is a gift of God," his foster sister and guardian says.[7]

Another example is described by Dr. Kenneth Vaux, professor of ethics in medicine at the University of Illinois at Chicago Health Sciences Center. He relates a conversation he had with a 12-year-old girl who has spina bifida. "She said to me, 'Ken, I know why I was born this way.' I said, 'Oh, no.' Well, she pulled those big old arm braces of hers up and started playing the harp, with those marvelous arms and fingers that spina bifida individuals develop. It brought tears to my eyes, because she had discovered something. She had discovered a gift, a power. She could say, it's okay that I'm this way."[8]

Although Leslie Lemke and this girl are exceptional cases, they are reminders not to underestimate the handicapped person's ability to contribute—whether it's with a hug, a smile, or a song. But even Lemke would never have done so if, when he was eight, his adoptive mother hadn't bought a piano and put his fingers onto the keys, helping him push them to make sounds.

Family Members Need God's Promises

Parents, who've spent endless hours in hospital waiting rooms, watching their child hurt without being able to make the pain go away, need promises from Scripture that they can integrate into their lives. The child also needs them for obvious reasons. These promises can direct their thoughts to God and provide assurance that they're not alone—that the Lord of the universe is with them through this trial and will enable them to cope. Here are some topics of encouragement, brief explanations, and references where they are found:

• *Grace*—God's kindness is available without limit, day by day, moment by moment: II Corinthians 12:9.

- *God's intervention*—Individuals need not feel oppressed by their circumstances, because, painful as they may be, our God is Lord and will work His sovereign will through them: Romans 8:28, 29.
- *Comfort*—The one who dwells in the reborn human spirit will soothe, console, and provide hope: II Corinthians 1:3, 4.
- *Deliverance*—God promises not necessarily to change circumstances but to be a refuge in the midst of them: All of Psalm 91, especially verses 1, 2.
- *Strength*—God has promised that His power will be available to cope with circumstances, just as it was for Steve and Pam Harris as they have had to endure stress each of the more than 2,700 times their son Matthew stopped breathing: Isaiah 40:28-31; 41:10.
- *Wisdom*—It's important that individuals be able to view their situation with understanding and be able to trust God to guide them when they have to make decisions: James 1:5.
- *Presence of the Holy Spirit*—Families often feel alone and frightened: John 14:16-18.
- *The Spirit's help in prayer*—Circumstances can be so confusing, individuals don't know how to pray: Romans 8:26, 27.
- *Peace*—Because of inherent limitations and an often uncertain future, handicapped children and their parents may struggle with fear and anxiety. The inner calm and tranquility they need is available in Christ: John 14:27; Philippians 4:4, 7.

Pastor Steve Harris assures parents of handicapped children that God faithfully keeps His promises. "There have been many times when I have literally felt the hands of God helping me through a situation I didn't think I could handle (such as my first Mother's Day sermon with Matthew still hospitalized)." He says it was God who enabled him to go on with his work while he was hurting. Both he and the congregation he serves have personally experienced the truth of the verse written on a plaque given to the family on the birth of their precious son:

Matthew

Gift of the Lord

"The Lord is good; a stronghold
in the day of trouble. He knows
those who take refuge in Him."

from Nahum 1:7

CHAPTER SEVEN

THE LAW AND THE HANDICAPPED CHILD

DRAMATIC PROGRESS HAS BEEN MADE IN RECENT YEARS assuring that equal opportunities are available for all people—especially the disabled. Legislation has been a large contributor to this progress.

Public Law 94-142—The Education for All Handicapped Children Act

These days, a handicapped child has greater opportunity than ever to develop his or her potential. One reason for this is Public Law 94-142.

"PL 94-142 is the dream law that changed the school world for millions of American children and their families," applauds Joyce Slayton Mitchell in *Taking on the World*.[1] Wherever you go these days, you'll hear parents cheering with her.

Why is that, you ask? Public Law 94-142 is the Education for All Handicapped Children Act passed by Congress in 1975. This law guarantees free and appropriate education (through elementary and high school) in the least restrictive environment possible for children with disabilities. It says:

This law requires the state to establish . . . procedures to assure that, to the maximum extent appropriate, handicapped children, including children in public or private institutions or other care facilities, are educated with children who are not handicapped and that special classes, separate schooling, or other removal of handicapped children from the regular educational environment occurs only when the nature and severity of the handicap is such that education in regular classes with the use of supplementary aids and services cannot be achieved satisfactorily.[2]

As Sol Gordon reported in *One Miracle at a Time*, before PL 94-142, of the approximately eight million disabled children in the U.S. between the ages of 3-21, over one million were excluded from the public school system. Now, all children are to be served.

Judith D. Singer, writing in *The Educational Digest*, calls this law "a handicapped children's Bill of Rights."[3] To a parent this means that their child, regardless of the type or severity of the handicap, is afforded an opportunity for the same educational privileges as children without disabilities. He or she is not to be sequestered from so-called "normal" children but are to be mainstreamed in whatever ways are appropriate.

Each individual state in its own educational districts is to put this law into practice. How this is being done varies widely from place to place. So does interpretation of key words in that law, such as *appropriate* and *least restrictive environment*. For that reason, the child's parents or caretakers need to be encouraged to act as advocates on their child's behalf.

Many parents are pleased with the education their child is receiving and feel that school districts are trying to comply with PL 94-142. Others are less satisfied. For this reason parents must be aware of the rights of their child and remain actively involved with the school in the education process.

In order for a counselor or helper to encourage parents in doing this, he or she needs to know what the family has been guaranteed under the law. Here are some particulars:

- Every child has a right to be evaluated before they are placed in special education. Parents obtain this evaluation by giving a written request that the child be tested to the school principal or the special education director; then they should receive a written report containing the conclusions and recommendations of the evaluation team. (The child is to be tested by more than one specialist.) If parents do not agree with the evaluation, they have a right to obtain independent testing for which the school district may reimburse them. A list of qualified testers must be provided by the local school district. Dr. Charlotte Thompson urges parents to see that testing is done by a qualified expert, such as a psychologist trained in testing handicapped children. Parents also have the right to withhold permission to have their child tested. Reevaluation is to be done every three years.

- Parents have the right to an Individual Education Program (IEP), a written agreement between them and the school stating the special education services that will be furnished for their child. Parents and child have a right to participate in these annual planning meetings. The IEP is to provide services for

100

individual needs and to include transportation, counseling, medical services, physical and speech therapy, etc.

• Every child has the right to be placed in a school as close to home and in the least restrictive environment possible. He or she must be placed immediately after the IEP is written. Parents are part of the committee that decides where schooling will take place.

• Parents have the right to see and receive copies of their child's records, to restrict permission for no one other than the school or public agencies to use the information in those records, and to have them explained by a qualified professional.

• If the needs of the child are not being met, parents have the right to request a "due process" hearing within 45 days of that request and, if they lose, to appeal that decision. They also have a right to bring a lawsuit against the school district if they fail to prevail in the hearing and appeals process.

If the child is placed in a private school by the state or local education system, this is done at no cost to the parent. Further information on special educational programs in specific locations can be obtained by contacting state, county or local educational offices.[4]

Educational options which are available in many locations include schools devoted to children with a particular disability such as deafness; special education classes in the local school so the child can spend time in the regular classroom as well; and attendance in a regular classroom with adaptive equipment available, perhaps including someone to assist in special individual needs.

Children whose handicaps prevent them from attending school can be taught at home by a tutor. In these situations parents would have to contact the local school system to make arrangements for a "homebound" tutor.

"Dumping" a disabled child into public school without proper provisions, precautions, and assistance (such as tutors) can have disastrous results.

That's what happened to Tina.

Blind and brain damaged, Tina had been attending a state school for the blind. When she was suddenly and without preparation transferred to public school, Tina became confused, disoriented, and miserable. One day she was even knocked down a flight of stairs by students rushing to class.

That incident sent Tina's mother to school to talk to the principal. "Something had to be done," she said. Together, they came up with alternatives. Tina would be let out of class early to provide extra time for her to pass to the next class. She would also be assigned a "buddy" who would walk with her.

These ideas worked. A few years later, a well-adjusted Tina walked across the platform to receive her high school diploma.

Sydney Griffin, the parent of a daughter with cerebral palsy, described her experiences when it came time for Vanessa to go to school. Griffin visited four schools before she found one she felt was right for her daughter. "The administrators had all meant well. . . . They saw Vanessa as a cerebral palsy child. She couldn't walk or use her right hand, and her vocabulary consisted of only about 20 words. They emphasized her disability. But I knew my daughter. I recognized her abilities."[5]

After visiting a special school for disabled children recommended by the administrators, Griffin asked about other options. She then visited three special education programs for preschoolers. She settled on the one in which the teacher's ability was most impressive. After three months, Vanessa was walking without help; at the end of the first school year, her vocabulary was 3 times what it had been.

Section 504 of the Rehabilitation Act of 1973

This act was another important landmark for handicapped children. It forbids discrimination in publicly funded services and programs against persons with disabilities.

Parents need to know that it means schools are required to be accessible to handicapped people—with ramps for those in wheelchairs and desks at which a disabled child can work comfortably. In other words, schools are to be barrier-free.

Kate Hoffman, born without a right hand, says "Section 504 is a civil rights law. It protects our freedom to participate in all social institutions and services which receive certain kinds of federal money. . . . It has helped me realize that I am a creative and dignified human being."[6]

While federal law guarantees education to children of grade and high school age, it doesn't make provision for younger ones. As a result some states have enacted laws to provide early intervention for them. In Minnesota, for example, children under age five who are substantially developmentally delayed are now eligible for special services from birth. The family needs to investigate whether such programs are available in their state.

But education and its accompanying services are not all that federal law provides. Another important program that families should be aware of is the one for developmentally disabled people. It provides a variety of services, including diagnosis, evaluation and treatment of the condition, special living arrangements, job training, sheltered workshops, information services, and transportation. (Because these programs are administered by the state, they will vary from place to place.) Some specific programs include the following:

- *Project Head Start*—designed for children ages three to five. Among its services are medical, nutritional, and educational. Ten percent of the children enrolled in Head Start nationally must be handicapped, according to governmental funding stipulations.

- *Supplemental Security Income* (SSI)—additional monthly allotments available to families of children with disabilities whose income and assets are limited.

- *Medicaid* or *Medical Assistance Programs*—provide physical and related health services to families with low incomes. Eligibility requirements vary from state to state, but, generally, those who are receiving SSI, welfare, or other public assistance will qualify. (Medicaid isn't available in Arizona.)

- *Medicaid Supplemental Medical Care Assistance*—available to some families with higher incomes or where the child's medical expenses exceed a particular level.

- *Crippled Children's Services* (CCS)—provides medical and other related services for handicapped children from birth to age 21. All states must provide medical diagnosis and evaluation at no cost for all handicapped children. The Early Periodic Screening, Diagnosis and Treatment Program (EPSDT) determines whether children from low-income families require health care.

- *Vocational Rehabilitation*—available in every state, helps handicapped people become employable in a variety of ways, including providing financial assistance and training. Every handicapped young adult is evaluated individually and a course of action laid out. This plan may include providing special equipment like hearing aids, vocational counseling, college tuition, and job placement.

The law provides a variety of other kinds of services in different areas, such as residential services in family settings for those unable to reside in the community on their own, therapy, and visiting nurse's service. Once families have been helped to begin to investigate what is available in their area, they'll probably discover assistance they didn't know existed.

Human Rights—a New Issue

In addition to legal rights, handicapped children have human rights. Only recently has this become a topic of public discussion. Handicapped children need help and support in seeing that those rights—such as dignity, freedom from exploitation, oppression, isolation, and the pursuit of happiness—are protected.

In the past, it wasn't uncommon for children with disabilities to be hidden in back bedrooms of homes—homes where embarrassment and shame was stronger than love. These children became men and women who were never able to develop their potentials. They were fed, watered, and left to rock or stare—or worse.

That is changing. Children in wheelchairs are everywhere these days. Deaf children sign to their parents as they ride the bus together; mentally impaired people ride beside us to and from their jobs in sheltered workshops. They sit in our church sanctuaries.

But the transition from back bedroom to society's mainstream is by no means complete. Flagrant violation of the human rights of handicapped children still takes place. Disabled people, for example, are some of the most susceptible to sexual abuse.

By assisting just one family, a Christian helper can make a contribution that can have a rippling effect in society.

Here is a summary of ways to do that:

- Work to bring parents and relatives to accept their child.
- Encourage them to provide their child with the best possible environment in which to grow.
- Direct the family to resources that will promote physical mental and emotional development of the child.
- Help families discover what the law provides for these children and encourage them to act as advocates on their child's behalf.
- When necessary, make sure the child is protected from abuses.
- Show parents how to locate resources for adaptive equipment, medical and financial assistance, etc., so the child has the best

chance to be all he or she can be.

- Promote the concept that handicapped are persons of worth, created in the image of God—individuals in whom He can live and through whom He can reveal Himself.
- If possible, remain involved and available as a counselor as the child and family enter new life stages that are stressful.
- Cultivate the same rapport with handicapped children and youth that you would with others in the church.
- See that the child learns about the Gospel in a way he or she can understand, that the child experiences the love of God through His Body, the Church, and that the child is nurtured toward maturity in Christ and given opportunities to cultivate abilities and make contributions in the church.

By participating in the life of the family of one handicapped child, a counselor or pastor can make a tough life easier. Carl Hershey, a youth who is a hemophiliac, says, "If I had a magic wand, I would make people where they wouldn't have any problems, and all the world would be one big happy family, and everybody would be a person to each other, and nobody would have hangups or nothing. If someone had a problem, you know, like being in a wheelchair and stuff, I'd make them just be a normal person, where they could walk and run and do whatever they wanted."[7]

There are no magic wands. But there is the love of God, incarnate in His people.

Advocate. A volunteer who speaks in support of a disabled person and is their friend.

Autism. A developmental disability that begins in early childhood and is characterized by communication and behavior disorders.

Cerebral palsy. A group of disabling conditions caused by damage to the central nervous system that often results in lack of muscle control and may be accompanied by other conditions.

Cleft palate. Birth defect in which the roof of the mouth does not close; defect may also involve the upper lip and nose; correctable with surgery.

Deinstitutionalization. Removing a handicapped individual from a care facility to a group home or other residence in the community.

Developmental disability. Physical and mental disabilities that begin before 21 years of age, continue indefinitely, and are of significant severity.

Down's syndrome. A chromosomal abnormality that results in mental retardation and other characteristics.

Epilepsy. A disorder marked by disturbed electrical rhythms in the brain works resulting in one or more kinds of seizures.

Hearing impairment. Ranges from hearing loss to complete deafness.

Hemophilia. A hereditary condition in which blood fails to clot quickly enough, causing uncontrollable bleeding, even from small cuts.

Learning disabilities. Covers a variety of syndromes, such as dyslexia and perceptual handicaps. Affects ability to understand and use language.

Microcephalus. Abnormally small cranium.

Muscular dystrophy. A group of disorders characterized by the wasting away of muscles.

Multiple handicapped. More than one handicap, such as blindness and deafness. May also be called *severe handicap* which indicates an intense degree of a condition.

Mental retardation. Below average, general intellectual functioning. Includes Down syndrome.

Orthopedically impaired. Impairment or absence of bones and joints that may be congenital or the result of trauma or other disease.

Seizure. An episode of altered brain activity which may be sudden and brief or may continue for extended periods of time. May include loss or clouding of consciousness and mild or exaggerated movements.

Spina bifida. Incomplete closure of the spinal column that may cause muscle weakness or paralysis below the cleft, loss of sensation below the cleft, and loss of bowel and bladder control. May also result in hydrocephalus, an accumulation of fluid on the brain. May include learning problems.

Spinal cord injury. Injury to the spinal cord causing paralysis from the point of injury downward. May also result from a tumor on the spinal cord.

Residential care facility. Types of group homes for handicapped that provide care. May include numerous other services.

Respite care. Short-term care for persons with handicaps in order to give parents and guardians relief and rest.

Sheltered workshops. Facilities that provide vocational training and employment for individuals with disabilities.

Speech and language impairments. Includes inability to speak fluently, to articulate, to form words.

Visual impairment. Includes low vision (limited distance vision), minimal vision (light perception), and absence of vision.

This is not a complete list of terms. Others can be found in resources listed in the bibliography.

Chapter One

1. Jerry Adler, "Every Parent's Nightmare," in *Newsweek*, March 16, 1987, p. 64.

2. *Webster's New World Dictionary of the American Language*, (G. & C. Merriam Co., 1977).

3. Joyce S. Mitchell, *Taking on the World* (Harcourt Brace Jovanovich, New York, 1982), p. xiii.

4. Patty McGill Smith, "You Are Not Alone: For Parents When They Learn That Their Child Has a Handicap," (National Information Center for Children and Youth, 1984).

5. Judith Joggis, *The Disabled and Their Parents* (Charles B. Slack, 1975), p. 151.

6. Charlotte E. Thompson, *Raising a Handicapped Child* (William Morrow and Co., Inc., 1986), p. 14.

7. Ibid., p. 20.

8. James McAlister, "Is Hers a Life Worth Living?" in *Moody Monthly*, October, 1982, p. 77.

Chapter Four

1. Elain Fein, "Should We Keep Our Baby?" in *Woman's Day*, November 20, 1987, p. 68.

2. Martha Moraghan Jablow, *Cara* (Temple University Press, 1982), p. 13.

3. "The Littlest Victims," in *Ladies' Home Journal*, September, 1985, p. 11.

4. Donald Peake, "Their Rightful Place," in *The Alliance Witness*, November 21, 1984, p. 8.

5. Gary R. Collins, Ph.D., *Christian Counseling* (Word Books, 1980), p. 457.

6. Leo Buscaglia, *The Disabled and Their Parents: a Counseling Challenge* (Charles B. Slack, Inc., 1975), pp. 277, 278.

7. Beatrice A. Wright, *Physical Disability—A Psychological Approach* (Harper & Row, 1960), p. 109.
8. Caren Ferris, *A Hug Just Isn't Enough* (Gallaudet College Press). p. 8.
9. Matthew Linn, S.J., Dennis Linn, S.J., *Healing Life's Hurts: Healing Memories through Five Stages of Forgiveness* (Paulist Press, 1978) p. 91
10. Ira T. Tanner, *The Gift of Grief: Healing the Pain of Everyday Losses* (Hawthorne Books, 1976).
11. Richard P. Walters, *Anger: Yours and Mine and What to Do About It* (Zondervan, 1981), p. 77.
12. Ibid., p. 80.
13. Linn, *Healing Life's Hurts,* pp. 128, 129.
14. Ibid., p. 136.
15. Gary R. Collins, Ph.D., *Christian Counseling* (Word Books, 1980), pp. 124, 125.
16. Adler, *Newsweek,* p. 60.
17. Charlotte E. Thompson, MD, *Raising a Handicapped Child* (William Morrow and Co., Inc., 1986) p. 187.

Chapter Five

1. Irving R. Dickman and Sol Gordon, *Getting Help for a Disabled Child—Advice from Parents* (Public Affairs Committee, Inc., 1983), pp. 11, 12.
2. Bette M. Ross, *Our Special Child* (Walker, 1981), pp. 56-65.
3. Joyce S. Mitchell, *Taking on the World* (Harcourt Brace Jovanovich, 1982), p. 51.
4. Carol Kramer, "Sometimes We Feel We're the Luckiest People Alive," in *McCalls,* February, 1985, p. 54.
5. Ross, *Our Special Child,* p. 51.

Chapter Six

1. Steve Harris, "When the Pastor Is Hurting," in *Leadership,* Spring, 1985, p. 110.
2. Ibid., p. 112.
3. Joni Eareckson and Steve Estes, *A Step Further* (Zondervan, 1978), pp. 46, 55, 157.
4. C. S. Lewis, *The Problem of Pain* (Macmillan Co., 1962), p. 110.
5. Ibid., p. 34.

6. Steven Baer, "Should Imperfect Infants Survive?" in *National Review*, September 2, 1983, pp. 1069, 1093.
7. Lewis H. Arends, Jr., "Handicapped 'Miracle Man' in Concert," in *Statesman Journal*, January 26, 1986.
8. "Can God Make Your Pain Go Away?" in *U.S. Catholic*, August, 1984, p. 8.
9. Harris, *Leadership*, p. 113.

Chapter Seven

1. Joyce S. Mitchell, *Taking on the World*, (Harcourt Brace Jovanovich, 1982), p. 32.
2. *Preparation for Life: A Manual for Parents on the Least Restrictive Environment, Vol. II*, prepared for the Technical Assistance for Parents Programs (Federation for Children with Special Needs and the Center on Human Policy, 20 USC 1412 5 B), p. 12.
3. Judith D. Singer, "Educating Handicapped Children—10 Years of PL 94-142," in *The Educational Digest*, December, 1985, p. 47.
4. Some information in this chapter is based on resources published by the Oregon Association for Children and Adults with Learning Disabilities and *The Pocket Guide to Federal Help for the Disabled Person.*
5. Sydney J. Griffin, "Special Child, Special Class," in *The American Baby*, November, 1986, p. 58.
6. William Roth, *The Handicapped Speak*. (McFarland & Co.), p. 35.
7. Ibid., p. 96.

Books on Disabilities and Children

Ayrault, Evelyn West, 1964. *You Can Raise Your Handicapped Child*. New York: G. P. Putnam's Sons. General, helpful information.

Batshaw, Mark L., 1981. *Children with Handicaps: A Medical Primer*. Baltimore, MD: Paul H. Brookes, Publishers. Facts regarding children who are born with developmental disabilities.

Cruzie, Kathleen, 1982. *Disabled? Yes; Defeated? No*. Englewood Cliffs, NJ: Spectrum Books/Prentice Hall. Resources and ideas for disabled people, their families, and others.

Darling, Rosalyn B., and Darling, Jon, 1982. *Children Who Are Different*. St Louis: C. V. Mosby Co. Sociologists' insights for professionals and others.

Dickman, Irving R., and Gordon, Sol, 1985. *One Miracle at a Time: How to Get Help for Your Disabled Child—From the Experience of Other Parents*. New York: Simon and Schuster.

Doyle, Phillis B., et al, 1979. *Helping the Severely Handicapped Child: A Guide for Parents and Teachers*. New York: Thomas Y. Crowell. Helps to obtain public education and solve other problems that come up in the daily lives of families with severely disabled children.

Eareckson, Joni and Estes, Steve, 1978. *A Step Further*. Grand Rapids, MI: Zondervan. Joni talks about suffering.

Ferris, Caren. *A Hug Just Isn't Enough*. Washington, DC: Gallaudet College Press. Statements by parents about their children's deafness. Provides insights.

Heslinga, K.; Schellen, A. M. C. M.; and Verkuyl, A., 1974. *Not Made of Stone—The Sexual Problems of Handicapped People*. Springfield, IL.: Charles C. Thomas Co.

Kubler-Ross, Elisabeth, 1974. *Questions and Answers on Death and Dying*. New York: MacMillan Publishing Co., Inc. Popular book on the grief process. Principles apply to acceptance of a child's handicaps.

Mitchell, Joyce Slayton, 1980. *See Me More Clearly.* New York: Harcourt Brace Jovanovich. Career and life planning for teens with physical disabilities.

Mitchell, Joyce Slayton, 1982. *Taking on the World.* New York: Harcourt Brace Jovanovich. How to overcome problems in family life, medical care, education, church, vocation, and government as they relate to disabled people.

National Health Committee, compiler, 1976. *The Killers and Cripplers.* New York: David McKay Co., Inc. Brief explanations of a variety of handicaps. Statistics may be outdated, but worth reading for still applicable information.

Ohsberg, Oliver H., 1982. *The Church and Persons with Handicaps.* Scottdale, PA: Herald Press. Includes Biblical insights as well as facts about the handicapped.

Oosterveen, Gerald, and Cook, Bruce L., 1983. *Serving Mentally Impaired People: A Resource Guide for Pastors and Church Workers.* Elgin, IL: David C. Cook Publishing Co. Includes basic information, plus data on life-style, theology, history, and psychology of the mentally impaired.

Roberts, Nancy, 1981. *Help for Parents of a Handicapped Child.* St. Louis, MO: Concordia Publishing House.

Russell, Mark L., 1983. *Alternatives: A Family Guide to Legal and Financial Planning for the Disabled.* Evanston, IL: First Publications. How care can be provided when a disabled child becomes an adult.

Thompson, Charlotte E., M.D., 1986. *Raising a Handicapped Child.* New York: Morrow. A comprehensive, helpful guide for parents of the physically disabled child.

Towns, E., and Groff, R. L., 1972. *Successful Ministry to the Retarded.* Chicago: Moody Press.

Paterson, George W., 1975. *Helping Your Handicapped Child.* Minneapolis: Augsburg Publishing House. Shows how parents can meet their disabled child's needs and gain strength through faith.

Wedemeyer, A., 1975. *Creative Ideas for Teaching Exceptional Children.* Denver: Love Publishing Co.

Wheeler, Bonnie, 1980. *Of Braces and Blessings.* New York: Christian Herald Books. The story of a couple whose three children had serious health problems, how God helped them cope, and how He led them to adopt three more such children.

Wheeler, Bonnie, 1983. *Challenged Parenting*. Ventura, CA: Regal Books. Helps for parents of handicapped children. Written by the mother of six "challenged" children, three biological and three adopted.

Wilke, Harold H., 1980. *Creating the Caring Congregation*. Nashville: Abingdon Press. Helps leaders and laypeople include handicapped people as part of the church.

Books on Counseling

Buscaglia, Leo, Ph.D., 1975. *The Disabled and Their Parents: A Counseling Challenge*. Thorofare, NJ: Slack, Inc. A guide to help professionals work with disabled people and their families.

Collins, Gary R., Ph.D., 1980. *Christian Counseling*. Waco, TX: Word Books. A comprehensive guide to counseling which includes topics pertinent to families with handicapped children.

Books for Siblings

Brothers and sisters of the handicapped child, as well as other children, will benefit by reading books about peers who are disabled. See the children's section of your library for additional titles.

Greenfield, Eloise, and Revis, Alesia, 1981. Drawings by Ford, George; photography by Bond, Sandra. *Alesia*. New York: Philomel Books. True story of a girl disabled at nine years of age, told in diary fashion.

Klein, Gerda, *The Blue Rose*, 1974. New York: Laurence Hill. Explains why a girl named Jenny is different from other girls, and why she needs more love and understanding.

Rosenberg, Maxine, 1983. Photography by Anacona, George. *My Friend Leslie*. New York: Lothrop, Lee, and Shepard Books. A picture and story book about a multihandicapped child.

Tada, Joni Eareckson, 1988. *Darcy*. Elgin, IL: David C. Cook Publishing Co. Joni uses fiction to convey the message of acceptance and love through this first-person story of a twelve-year-old girl in a wheelchair. Reading level: ages ten through twelve.

Tada, Joni Eareckson, 1988. *Ryan and the Circus Wheels*. Ryan's day at the circus with his class seems spoiled when his wheelchair-bound sister comes along as "room mother." But Ryan's embarrassment turns into a prayer for help when he gets lost. Reading level: ages four through seven.

Tada, Joni Eareckson, 1987. *Meet My Friends*. Elgin, IL: David C. Cook Publishing Co. Joni writes about three special young friends who, like herself, have overcome disabilities. The book helps children see that these three kids are first of all people like themselves. Reading level: ages eight through ten.

For Information on a Disabled Child's Rights

American Coalition of Citizens with Disabilities, 1200 15th St. N.W., Washington, DC 20036

The Children's Defense Fund, 122 C Street N.W., Washington, DC 20001

Literature from Federal Agencies

The following three booklets are available for a nominal charge from Public Affairs Pamphlets, 381 Park Avenue South, N.Y., NY 10016.

#473: "Living with Blindness" by Irving R. Dickman, 28 pp.

#504: "Helping the Handicapped Teenager Mature" by Evelyn West Ayrault, 28 pp.

#615: "Getting Help for a Disabled Child—Advice from Parents" by Irving R. Dickman and Sol Gordon, 28 pp.

The following three reference circulars are available from the National Library Service for the Blind and Physically Handicapped, The Library of Congress, Washington, DC 20542:

#84-2: "Building a Library Collection on Blindness and Physical Handicaps: Basic Materials and Resources," 52 pp. A valuable bibliography.

#84-5: "Parents' Guide to the Development of Preschool Handicapped Children: Resources and Services," 25 pp. A list of recordings and educational toys for preschool handicapped children, plus a selected bibliography of books, periodicals, and national organizations of interest to parents.

#86-1: "Selected Readings for Parents of Preschool Handicapped Children," 10 pp. A listing of books and periodicals of interest to parents of disabled children.

The following material is available from the U.S. Department of Education, Washington, DC 20202:

#E85-22002: "Pocket Guide to Help for the Disabled Person."

Periodicals

The Exceptional Parent, 296 Boylston Street, Third Floor, Boston, MA 02116. Published six times a year. Contains articles that cover the spectrum of caring for a child who has a disability.

National Information Clearinghouse

The National Information Center for Handicapped Children and Youth (NICHCY) is a national clearinghouse that offers free information packets about disabilities, answers specific questions, and makes referrals to other organizations. Write NICHCY, P.O. Box 1492, Washington DC 20013. Or call (703) 522-3332. NICHCY is a good place to start when looking for information.

Curriculum for Disabled Children

The Friendship series, a Christian education program to meet the needs of persons with mental impairments, is available from the David C. Cook Publishing Co., 850 N. Grove Ave., Elgin, IL 60120.

Concordia Publishing House (3558 S. Jefferson Ave., St. Louis, MO 63118) publishes Christian education materials for the developmentally disabled as well as curriculum for the hearing impaired.

The *Happy Time* course, a curriculum for mentally handicapped students, is available from Scripture Press Publications, 1825 College Ave., Wheaton, IL 60187.

The Sunday School Board of the Southern Baptist Convention (127 Ninth Ave. N., Nashville, TN 37234) publishes resources for teaching deaf children.

Joni and Friends (28720 Canwood St., P.O. Box 3333, Agoura Hills, CA 91301) distributes books, records, video, and other educational material which help able-bodied children relate to the disabled.

A two-part children's video curriculum, *Joni in Let's Be Friends and Meet My Friends,* is available from the David C. Cook Publishing Co. The video features Joni Eareckson and her husband Ken. The two sessions encourage disabled children to see themselves as special to God, and lead able-bodied kids to form friendships with disabled people. A corresponding leader's guide is available.

Vocational Rehabilitation

American Occupational Therapy Association, 1383 Piccard Drive, Rockville, MD 20850

Department of Education, Rehabilitation Services Administration, 330 C Street S.W., Washington, DC 20202

Goodwill Industries of America, 9200 Wisconsin Avenue, Washington, DC 20814

Rehabilitation Agencies

National Association of Rehabilitation Facilities, P.O. Box 17675, Washington, DC 20041

Department of Education, Special Education and Rehabilitative Services, 330 C Street S.W., Washington, DC 20202

Department of Health and Human Services, Administration on Developmental Disabilities, 200 Independence Ave, S.W., Washington, DC 20202

National Parent Organizations

Parentele, c/o Patricia Koerber, 5538 N. Pennsylvania Street, Indianapolis, IN 46220; or Elaine Clearfield, 310 S. Jersey St., Denver, CO 80224. Links members in a communication system; includes parents, professionals and service organizations.

Pilot Parents, c/o Keryn Paul, Omaha Association for Retarded Citizens, 3610 Dodge, Omaha, NE 68131. Trains parents to help other parents.

National Parent CHAIN, 515 W. Giles Lane, Peoria, IL 60614. Links parents and professional groups.

The Parent to Parent National Project, University Affiliated Program, University of Georgia, 850 College Station Rd., Athens, GA 30610. Provides information and support to parents of newborn and newly diagnosed children with disabilities.

PACER Center, Inc., 4826 Chicago Ave., Minneapolis, MN 55417. A source of information for parents of children and youth with any type of disability.

Organizations Helping Children with All Disabilities

The National Easter Seal Society, 2023 W. Ogden Ave., Chicago, IL 60612. Provides physical, occupational and speech/language therapies, vocational evaluation and training, camping, recreation, psychological counseling, equipment, informational referral, and enabling fund. Approximately 200 state and local societies.

Shriners Hospitals for Crippled Children, 2900 Rocky Point Drive, Tampa, FL 33607. Nineteen orthopedic hospitals and three burn institutes that offer care and treatment to children up to age 18 free of charge—if, in the opinion of the hospital's chief of staff, there is a reasonable possibility that treatment will benefit the child and that treatment at another facility would place a financial burden on the patient's family or guardian.

Public Agencies

The National Information Center for Handicapped Children and Youth (NICHCY—see address under "National Information Clearinghouse" in this Bibliography) lists the following public agencies who are responsible for providing certain kinds of assistance to disabled people and their families. Upon request, NICHCY will send a list of the names and addresses of agencies in your state. They recommend the local school district as one of the best resources.

Your state department of education answers questions on how to get special education services in your state.

The office of state coordinator of vocational education for handicapped students can tell you what programs are in existence, how funds are being used, and what new programs are planned.

State mental health agencies. Their functions vary from state to state. They should be able to direct you to local services.

Early Periodic Screening, Diagnosis, and Treatment Program (EPSDT) screens children to identify whether health care or related services are necessary. Available for Medicaid eligible children from birth to 21 years of age.

University affiliated facilities. To find those in your area that have programs for youth with handicaps, write The American Association of University Affiliated Facilities, Suite 813, 123 Massachusetts Ave., N.W., Washington DC 20005.

The state mental retardation agency provides information about services for persons with this disability.

Protection and advocacy services vary but generally provide information about education, health, residential services, and social services.

Crippled children's services help identify children with handicaps, diagnose their condition, and advise parents regarding treatment.

The state developmental disabilities agency, assisted by the federal government, provides diagnosis, evaluation, recreation, group homes, information, referral, social services, advocacy, and protection.

The state vocational rehabilitation agency provides medical, therapeutic, counseling, educational, training, and other services to prepare people with handicaps for work. The state will direct you to the nearest rehabilitation office.

National Organizations Helping Those with Specific Disabilities

The following organizations provide some, but not necessary all, of the following: research, medical care, education of professionals, influence of public policy, parent support, help in starting local support groups, job placement, newsletters, and publications lists.

American Ministries to the Deaf, 7564 Brown's Mill Rd., Kauffman Station, Chamersburg, PA 17201 (Bible correspondence school for deaf and deaf/blind, Bible teaching, visual aids).

Alexander Graham Bell Association for the Deaf, 3417 Volta Place, N.W., Washington, DC 20007. Phone: (202) 337-5220.

American Society for Deaf Children, 814 Thayer Ave., Silver Springs, MD 20910. Phone: (301) 585-5400.

Association for Retarded Citizens, 2501 Ave. J., Arlington, TX 76006. Phone: (817) 640-0204.

Autism: NSAC, 1234 Massachusetts Ave., N.W., Suite 1017, Washington, DC 20005. Phone: (202) 783-0125.

Cystic Fibrosis Foundation, 6000 Executive Blvd., Suite 309, Rockville, MD 20852. Phone: (301) 881-9130.

Epilepsy Foundation of America, 1419 Street, N.W., Washington, DC 20005.

March of Dimes Birth Defects Foundation, 1275 Mamaroneck Ave., White Plains, NY 10605. Phone: (914) 428-7100.

Muscular Dystrophy Association, 810 Seventh Ave., New York, NY 10019. Phone: (212) 586-0808.

National Association for the Visually Handicapped, 305 East

24th Street, 17-C, New York, NY 10010. Phone: (212) 889-3141.

National Down's Syndrome Congress, 1800 Dempster Rd., Park Ridge, IL 60608-1146. Phone: (312) 823-7750; or 1-800-232-NDSC outside Illinois.

National Federation of the Blind, P.O. Box 11185, Kansas City, KS 66111.

National Organization for Rare Disorders, P.O. Box 8923, New Fairfield, CT 06812.

National Paraplegia Association, 333 N. Michigan Ave, Chicago, IL 60601.

John Tracy Clinics (for the hearing impaired), 806 West Adams Boulevard, Los Angeles, CA 90007. Phone: (213) 748-5481.